Menstruation Now

WHAT DOES BLOOD PERFORM?

edited by Berkeley Kaite

DEMETER

Menstruation Now
What does blood perform?
Edited by Berkeley Kaite

Copyright © 2019 Demeter Press

Demeter Press
140 Holland Street West
P. O. Box 13022
Bradford, ON L3Z 2Y5
Tel: (905) 775-9089
Email: info@demeterpress.org
Website: www.demeterpress.org

Demeter Press logo based on the sculpture "Demeter" by Maria-Luise Bodirsky www.keramik-atelier.bodirsky.de

Printed and Bound in Canada

Front cover image: Untitled (from the Flower project, part one), Anna Volpi.
Front cover artwork: Michelle Pirovich
Typesetting: Michelle Pirovich

Library and Archives Canada Cataloguing in Publication
Title: Menstruation now : what does blood perform?
Editor: Berkeley Kaite.
Names: Kaite, Berkeley, editor.
Description: Includes bibliographical references.
Identifiers: Canadiana 20190066792 | ISBN 9781772581881 (softcover)
Subjects: LCSH: Menstruation—Social aspects. | LCSH: Menstrual cycle—Social aspects. | LCSH: Menstruation in literature. | LCSH: Menstruation in motion pictures. | LCSH: Menstruation on television.
Classification: LCC GN484.38 .M46 2019 | DDC 612.6/62—dc23

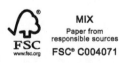

MIX
Paper from
responsible sources
FSC
www.fsc.org   FSC® C004071

I would like to acknowledge and thank Andrea O'Reilly for creating and sustaining Demeter Press and May Friedman for her work as project mentor. I am grateful for the expert and generous editorial skills of Jesse O'Reilly-Conlin. Thanks also to the reviewers of the manuscript for their helpful comments and feedback and to the contributors with whom it was a pleasure to work.

Contents

Introduction

Berkeley Kaite

This volume brings together textual analyses of different sites of menstrual performance. That is to say, each essay addresses menstrual blood not as an obdurate reality but as a sign with multiple connotations. Blood is a fluid. However, it is also meta-phorically fluid: blood is not only one thing but is "volatile" (Grosz) in its leakiness and, thus, in its ability to threaten boundaries, borders, and binaries.

Blood itself signifies differently depending on its embodied contexts. Receive a paper cut and you'll lick the blood off your finger. However, Germaine Greer asks in *The Female Eunuch* (1970), "if you think you are emancipated, you might consider the idea of tasting your menstrual blood—if it makes you sick, you've a long way to go, baby" (57). Note Greer's appropriation of 1970s feminist rhetoric. "Eman-cipation" belongs to second-wave discourses of liberation, freedom, and unrestraint of all kinds. In addition, commerce also belongs to the discourse of emancipation. Greer paraphrases the caption from a print ad for a cigarette marketed for women, Virginia Slims. In a nod to equality of the sexes, the cigarette was designed for the female and feminine consumer. It's slender; size matters. This series of ads featured comparisons between the trapped life of a nineteenth- or early-twentieth-century woman—who had to hide her cigarettes in her garter—and her modern counterpart, who can now smoke in public. The accompanying slogan is "you've come a long way, baby." Here, Greer wants to foreground a feminist appreciation of menstrual blood and to re-embody it through the invitation to taste it. But while that invitation acknowledges the idea of tasting menstrual blood may make you feel sick, it also urges that one get over that revulsion and try it. Greer suggests that embodiment, nausea in particular, and politics go together. Blood is never just one thing. It is performative.

The teenage ritual of cutting wrists and then mixing the blood through the rubbing together of those bleeding veins—and becoming blood sisters or brothers—is seen as benign and quaint, besides the hysteria surrounding the sharing of blood tainted by the HIV virus. Blood and belonging, blood ties—these words invoke the concept of the threshold, both the threshold of inside and outside and the body as threshold itself. The first binary of inside and outside means that blood of any kind exists inside the body but only after it exits—through a vein, a nose, a vagina—does it manifest as a sign. However, blood manifests not just one sign: blood is a signifier with several signifieds. A second binary posits the (presumed natural) body against culture. But blood helps us understand what Elizabeth Grosz argues is the body itself as a threshold—the "pivotal point" where cultural negotiations are both worked out and inscribed (23). The body, Grosz writes, "hovers perilously and undecidably at the pivotal point of binary pairs... neither—while also being both—the private or the public, self or other, natural or cultural, psychical or social, instinctual or learned, genetically or environmentally determined" (23). Grosz uses the Möbius strip as a model for the irreducibility of both the body's obdurate particulars and how they are represented and understood. The materials of embodiment and their cultural signification are inseparable and mutually inflected. Blood within this conception is a fluid that "attest(s) to the permeability of the body, its necessary dependence on an outside" (193). So while blood may seem to belong in the body, and in this case, a woman's body, when a cis-woman's uterine lining builds towards its monthly slow release, that fluid is charged with many disciplinary manoeuvres—material, linguistic, and symbolic. Although the average monthly flow consists of around a quarter of a cup of blood, contemporary ads for so-called feminine hygiene products invoke fluids as a feminine danger: overwhelming, uncontrollable, and massive in volume. In one recent ad for Always Infinity napkins, a tornado has morphed into a sea-blue cone of water and is poised to penetrate a sanitary napkin. The caption reads: "Your heavy days are going down" ("The Last"). In another ad for the same product, a napkin shaped as an umbrella shields another sanitary napkin. Raindrops are in the background. The caption says "Stay dry during downpours." A third ad for this brand mimics the graphics of a televised weather report with a "weekly flowcast" from Monday to

Friday ("25% spotting"; "50% moderate flow," etc.). An icon of a cloud with plump raindrops accompanies Thursday's "85% overnight flow" ("Case Studies"). Appropriately, the product is called "Always," as in you are always full of effluvia and which threatens a deluge without warning. Or, in the words of a contemporary ad for Stayfree, "The Hoover Dam has a better chance of springing a leak" ("Jack's Story").

The assumption is that cis-women are effluent and bloody emissions need a dam to staunch them—only a dam could do the job of stopping the relentless menstrual flow. The language used in this ad partakes of the discourse of emancipation Germaine Greer invoked in 1970, but it lands on the other side of a binary. Greer has her readers challenging ingrained feelings about their menstrual blood. Stayfree, on the other hand, has consumers challenging that blood itself. The language of defense (as the best offence) is invoked: the Stayfree maxi pad offers "leak protection ... with 18 anti-leak channels... an anti-leak core." It is a "revolutionary triple defense system." The mobilization of militaristic language and imagery goes beyond Greer's defiant entreaty though it isn't new. In the mid-1960s, Kotex, had "safety shields"— "2" of them ("Why Do?").

New Freedom "builds a better maxi" with "moisture-trap protection ... with 15 extra-absorbent layers that *trap* wetness in millions of tiny pockets." It is advertised as helping to "keep your clothes dry with a 3-sided stain shield" ("New Freedom"). The euphemistic moisture and wetness (i.e., blood) are equated with a stain. One's clothes are in need of protection. And although wetness is equated with the feminine, it is also aggressive in its assumptive capacity to tarnish the wearer's clothing and, to be sure, the wearer. Indeed, the Carefree ads from the early 1980s contain the slogan "for the fresh-dressed woman anytime!" ("1980"). The militaristic language—Carefree Essentials, a pantiliner, offers "double barrier protection"—finds its way in the slyly humorous short story by Alice Munro, "Chance." The heroine copes with her period while on a long train ride, and the narrator has her searching for "reinforcements."

Fortification is in the air—a militaristic stance whether against one's feelings, one's cultural norms, or one's body, especially its emissions. And here, in the name of fashion, a "fresh dressed" model is pictured in different outfits, always white. The clothes are fortified against immanent bloodstains. The products offer "protection" from the apparently massive monthly flow that requires a product to "pull" moisture in, "trap it deep, and hold it in millions of tiny pockets" ("1953 Kotex").

"Reinforcements" also refer to an emotional stance—the ever-ready position of defense against a surprise attack. But who might be surprised? The subject who bleeds, yes; but also, potentially, those around her. A most unwelcome surprise, the unruly feminine characterized by the capriciousness of blood (and vice versa) cannot be pinned down and is unstable in her effects. That volatility by its nature requires others be fortified against it/her. Reinforcement— invoking a boundary and a binary—is in the air. The subject herself is assumed to require protection against the inevitable menstrual flow and the presumption of its unsettling qualities. She is assumed to require reinforcement against the gaze of the other: a 1941 ad for Tampax has the caption "sharp eyes cannot tell" ("Sharp Eyes"). Others' eyes are the visual speculum to accompany this new kind of internal protection. The introduction of tampons corresponded with the mass participation of women in wage labour during the Second World War (Kaite). That is, with greater participation in public life and with greater interaction with other people came the issue of self-discipline—the impulse, if not need, to put oneself under surveillance. In 1942, a series of ads for Meds, "the modern tampon," features sketches of women engaged in jobs for the war effort—for example, a military nurse, an airplane mechanic, and a mechanic in military uniform changing the hubcap on a tire ("A Woman's Plight").

The effects of the circulation of the menstruating subject in public require its regulation (i.e., the internal surveillance of feminine blood). And although few would dispute the benefits and practicality of the tampon, it's the language that overdetermines the symbolic utility of these products. Meds contains a "safety centre," the notation of which is accompanied by a drawing of a tampon with an arrow pointing to the visually amplified interior, for effect. What/who is safe here? Whose safety is a concern, and from what? This anxiety is given sharper eyes in an ad from the 1970s for Demure, a vaginal deodorant, which describes the product as a necessity for women whose days involve meeting people, visiting places, and doing things. People, places, and things must be safe from feminine interiority and all that it contains, reveals, and obscures and all that it may potentially release:

it is a frightening unknown, a place to be filled with meanings (ellipses in other words).

Interiority, while literally silent, is metaphorically on the cusp of something. The enigma of this amorphous space is one half of the inside-outside binary; it is made to speak and to transgress its boundary in a variety of euphemisms. It's a cliché that menstruation and menstrual blood are taboo and subject to suppression and all manner of silences. However, the discursive construction of the menstruating subject is noisy—if one invokes a problematic binary of silence-noise— even if the noise is oblique, "told slant" (to borrow from Emily Dickinson), and employs verbal and visual euphemisms. Beginning in the late 1940s and continuing through to the early 1960s, Modess sanitary napkins had a campaign whose slogan contained only two words, phrased thusly: "Modess ... *because*." Note the rules of punctuation and style, all that might be packed into the ellipses and all that is suggested with the italics. And the word "because."

Ellipses contain all the words and assumed blood that strain to leak out—the humble period, three in a row because one is not enough, three periods that stand in for "the period." The ellipsis both abbreviates and expands: it aims for conciseness for it elides what is not said, and it invites imprecise filling in. "Ellipsis" comes from the Greek *elleipsis*, meaning defect or to fall short. In print, ellipses signify the intentional omission of words, a change of thought, a lapse in time, an incomplete construction. Grammatical ellipses both invite completion and deny that possibility at the same time. They take up (empty) space and time so there is a kind of free-flowing possibility of a conclusion. However, one falls short of a conclusion, as the three suggestive dots threaten to move madly off in all directions. Elusiveness is built into ellipses. It is a rather fitting convention when talking of blood, women, and, especially, feminine blood. Elizabeth Grosz reminds us of two things pertinent to this discussion: "Woman (uppercase and in the singular) remains philosophy's eternal enigma, its mysterious and inscrutable object" (4). And, following Luce Irigaray, the "disquiet" about blood as viscous, "half-formed, or the indeterminate has to do with the cultural unrepresentability of fluids within prevailing models of ontology, their implicit association with femininity, with maternity, with the corporeal, all elements sub-ordinated to the privilege of the self-identical, the one, the unified, the solid" (Grosz 195). Ellipses perfectly invoke the unrepresentable and the unsayable, not to say unspeakable. The ellipsis is both/and: things will not be uttered yet are strained to be heard. They say, *Use your imagination...*

Italics emphasize. They put an accent on the word by drawing attention to it. Originally used as an adjective to refer to something "of Italy," it is employed typically with foreign words and phrases or to set off a book title. Italics announce and command attention; putting the stress on a foreign word, a word that is spoken by others or that cannot be translated, suggests a *je ne sais quoi*. What cannot be translated with precision, and so is left in its original form and then italicized, suggests there is a struggle over meaning. Even though "because" is not a foreign phrase, it is laconic. What would it say if it could speak?

"Because" is a conjunction and a conjunction joins similar things together. Here, "because" joins a few things: the product's name (there is no image of the Modess napkin in the ad), a woman in beautiful repose, decked out in a high-end evening gown ("Because Modess"), the name itself connoting modesty. Yet what is modest here in this overt pose? Is it of a model in a studied display of wealth, leisure, and glamour? The name "Modess" and the word "modesty" both contain the root "mode" from its Indo-European origin, meaning "to measure." Embedded in the ad itself are the oblique features of an elliptical flow: though acknowledging the hidden presence of menstrual blood (even then the viewer does not know if this woman is supposed to be menstruating right now, in that dress, on this evening), its aesthetic details are finely and firmly in place, contained, still, frozen and measured. Blood here threatens impulsively to defile this image of immaculateness and is at the same time—indeed, due to its seeping and engulfing—held at bay, trapped by the product in waiting. Both/and are at play, much like the feminine figure that reveals the fraudulence of binary categories.

Gloria Steinem famously wrote that if men could menstruate they would "brag about how long and how much" (338). Instead, cis women menstruate, and that fact is dressed up in euphemism (*euphemizein*: to use words of good omen). Blood is everywhere, and it is not the case that its presence is suppressed, or only suppressed. Menstrual blood works its unruly way, along with the gendered body that is fashioned to contain it, into connotation. (Practically skipping denotation—

blood is viscous, but beyond that, euphemisms abound.) An ad series for Kotex from the 1950s contains the caption "not a shadow of a doubt" ("1953 Kotex"). Here too, as with the Modess ads mentioned above, the ideal model/consumer is featured in fashionable garb, and there are people in the background who look at her. She is in others' purview, and she knows it. In each ad, in small print, there is information about the clothes she is wearing, the designer, and the cost. This is a measured statement about fashion and the fashioning of the menstruating subject in public. What is in doubt here? What is the doubt that seems to hover precariously, invoked through its denial? A poetic discussion of this would playfully move between metaphors of certainty and hesitation. I will venture only to say that doubt is in the air. Doubt: from dubious which has "duo" and "to be" at its root. To be two is not to be the solid self-identical conceit of phallic masculinity. It is rather the more fickle, metaphorically multiple feminine.

That is also to say that in discourses of menstruation a binary of public display and suppression does not apply. The menstruating subject is constructed as noisy in her own way, always-already unruly. Many euphemisms are at play—the word blood is never used in advertisements—and it is their performative values that are addressed in *Menstruation Now.* Hence the subtitle, *What Does Blood Perform?*

What does it mean to speak of menstruation now? Not only one thing. "Performance" here is a pliable concept that moves beyond theatricality to embrace the enactment of meanings in language and image. If "performance" can imply the "restoration of behavior" (Schechner qtd. in Roach 46), then within its purview are the daily repetitions of acts, gestures, rituals, and utterances, both verbal and embodied, in and through which we engage. We have bodies, we live through our bodies, and we reproduce embodiment. And, we do this through these many instances of "twice-behaved behavior," which reveal the "materialization" of gendered norms (Butler 2) and, importantly, the way they can be re-materialized, re-performed, and performed again and, over time, differently. "Repeated, rehearsed, and above all recreated": no act or utterance is performed the same way twice and thus in "improvisatory behavioral space, memory reveals itself as imagination ... restored behavior ... represents an alternative and potentially contestatory form of knowledge—bodily knowledge, habit, custom" (Roach 46, 47). Blood in culture is repeated, rehearsed, and recreated, and it is embodied knowledge, custom, and habit. And perhaps more. It performs, and the chapters in this volume ask about those varied performative utterances. In so doing, they posit the potential for the re-materialization of representations of menstrual blood and, hence, their lived reality. Menstrual blood may invoke the need for a dam to staunch it, but the flow will continue and stories will reframe it. We may want to think of a sort of #BloodToo movement of its own and continue the conversation. Leakiness after all reveals the "arbitrariness of our dependency on binary opposition and neat categorization, and leads to a critique of the modern, masculine/ rational paradigm. Leaks dissolve bodily boundaries" (MacDonald 349). Shauna MacDonald suggests the resurrection of the threatening "revolution" in fluidity, and I offer the pan-language of advertising again with this example:

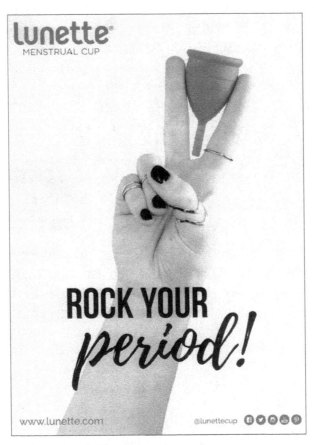

Reprinted with permission

The ad partakes of the literal and visual language of feminist insurrection, at least in its commercial dimension. I see this as congruent with the trajectories of different forms of "menstrual activism" (Bobel).

Active, from act, < *actus* means doing or moving. What the above discussion makes clear is that even though several stereotypes of women, femininity, and blood are still alive, the prevalence and volatility of the fluid, and as it intersects with feminist resistance, ensures its place among feminist activist platforms. The reclamation of menstruation speaks to the "new blood" in third-wave feminism as well as to the application of theory to practice, as Chris Bobel notes in her book of the same name, *New Blood: Third-Wave Feminism and the Politics of Menstruation*. Bobel underscores what "menstrual activism" does: it "seize[s] agentic menstrual consciousness from the docile, disciplined body and stimulate[s] new ways of knowing and being that neither shame nor silence" (41). The practical application of feminist theory to concrete objectives has taken many forms, among them: putting control of cis women's menstrual health into women's hands, critiquing products' safety, having an intersecting interest in the environment, and pushing back against profit-driven consumerist ethics (Bobel 42-65). So, for example, the emergence of alternatives to pads and tampons—sea sponges, diva cups, washable, and reusable cloth pads—is both out of concern for "environmental degradation" (Bobel 50) and a subversion of the feminine hygiene industry. The "alternative menstrual product market" (Bobel 60) is not the only form of activism. There are rituals based in spiritual practices and beliefs; there are interventionist tactics in zines, ad busting, culture jamming (e.g., the defacement of billboards), and boycotts (Bobel 97-134; Kissling 121). Sites and organizations—such as the online Museum of Menstruation and Women's Health and the Society for Menstrual Cycle Research— foreground and animate all manner of the material, medical, ideological, and cultural aspects to women's health and the menstrual cycle. Elizabeth Kissling refers to the "menstrual counterculture" in a chapter by the same name, and discusses the Museum of the Menovulatory Lifetime, which includes, among others, interactive exhibits and ideas about how to hold a "menstrual Monday" party (103-122). Lauren Rosewarne isolates some positive portrayals of menstruation in film and television—what she calls "bleeding out proud"—and attributes them to a "central achievement of feminism" (171). These "doings" are a kind of move-ment—activism in their own right—aspects of which are explored in the chapters that follow. Menstrual narratives are rarely quiet. Even while there may still be a "menstrual closet" (Fahs 1), Breanne Fahs joins Chris Bobel and others in noting the myriad "coherent, organized critiques and tactical interventions ... organic and informal modes of communication and connection ... showy and artistic public displays ... and more private and subtle shifts of thinking ... the culture of punk and anarchy alongside the do-it-yourself aesthetic " that go into the "raising [of] blood hell" (Fahs 3, 93). Fahs, as a therapist, has innovative chapters in *Out for Blood: Essays on Menstruation and Resistance* on her work with cis-gender and trans clients who, in disclosing the status of their menstrual cycles and feelings about menstrual blood, are "active" in examining the "diffuse boundaries between the public and private" (65).

Non-binary, trans, ethnic, and Indigenous: they are not equally represented in the media, nor are they, therefore, in *Menstruation Now*. There are crucial nuances to race, gender, ethnicity, and non-normative sexualities. However, Lauren Rosewarne adds a suggestive proviso to the lack of "minority" menstrual scenes in the media: "Through eschewing images of ethnic minorities—or, for that matter, *any* minority—in a menstrual narrative, the minority gets judged on her own merits and not with the added burden of a social taboo" (210). Blood in this instance, she concludes, would be a distraction. And as Chris Bobel points out, the movements involved in "alternative menstrual consciousness" (141) are frequently white yet also sometimes queer; their activists can still afford to engage in performances that do not threaten notions of "sexual respectability," as they do for women of colour (145ff.). *Menstruation Now* is not about the lived realities of the menstruating body—for example, the socioeconomic and cultural factors which intersect with race, ethnicity, religion, custom, and ritual. Most—many, not all—cis-women bleed, and so this kind of cultural "menstrual synchrony" (Rosewarne) is the shadow referent here. Menstrual blood respects age, but not much else, not class, race, religion, or ethnicity. So, what does blood symbolically activate? What does it perform?

Different media sites in *Menstruation Now* are interrogated for the ways in which menstrual blood is solicited to signify a variety of things. My chapter, "Bloody Jackie: How Menstrual Blood Speaks for Jacqueline Kennedy Onassis's Silence," wonders why some of Jackie's biographers mention the appearance of her menstrual blood on the morning of President Kennedy's assassination. Jackie is renowned for at least two things (before the marriage to "O"): her pink suit splattered with the blood of her husband and for never speaking publically about the assassination or, before that, her marriage to her presumed philanderer husband. Her menstrual blood, I argue, is a foil for that other orifice that would not speak. It is summoned as her body's uncensored utterance, especially unpredictable given all the secrets that remain of the assassination.

In "Who Is That 'She'? Narratives of Menstruation in the Terry Schiavo Case," Claire Horn analyzes the court transcripts of the legal battle that pitted Schiavo's husband against her parents. Schiavo had been in a persistent vegetative state for many years; her husband wanted her removed from life support so he could remarry, but her parents wanted her to remain alive. Evidence for what constitutes life and normal womanhood revolved around, among other things, the presence of Schiavo's menstrual cycle. Both parties referenced her blood, though differently, as silent testimony to her supposed, now forever unspoken, desires.

Laura Helen Marks uses the concept of the para-text (material unintended for the text but which makes its presence known) to analyze the phenomenon of menstrual blood in the pornographic film. "Period Porn: Menstrual Blood at the Margins" rescues blood from the apparent off-scene and suggests it is read, in its own right, as part of this ambiguously erotic, or erotically ambiguous genre of films. Here the unscripted moments of fluidity, and of feminine fluids, create an authentically embodied desire: blood here is not mimetic but seductive and like all seductions, powerfully imaginative, even fanciful.

Cayo Gamber analyzes of-the-moment advertisements, for example some of those on YouTube. In "'Changing the Conversation'" about Menstruation from 'Very Personally Yours' to #ItsNotMyPeriod: A Discursive Analysis of Menstrual Products and Advertisements," Gamber employs Kenneth Burke's ideas about what a "conversation" is to great effect. In charting some of the shifts in consciousness, rhetoric, political tone, and modes of address in the marketing of menstrual products over a few decades, Gamber isolates the honesty, humour, and passion at play and the necessity for keeping conversation-as-critical-inquiry as an ongoing enterprise (in real and virtual worlds).

Barbara Kutis looks at menstruation in art practice. In 1965, Shigeko Kabota put a brush in her underwear, dipped it in red paint, squatted, and painted menstrual strokes. Judy Chicago staged *Menstruation Bathroom* in the early 70s; it contained a wastebasket overflowing with bloody tampons. More recently, Sarah Maple in *Menstruate with Pride* and Rupi Kaur on Instagram are examples of menstrual displays with visibility and panache. Kutis's essay "The Contemporary Art of Menstruation: Embracing Taboos, Breaking Boundaries, and Making Art" uses Jacques Rancière's concept of "dissensus" to foreground how art may assault the senses and then reframe definitions of acceptability.

Peter Ohlin discusses Ingmar Bergman's film *Cries and Whispers*. In it, the main character Karin deliberately cuts her vagina with a shard of glass to mimic menstrual blood and get revenge on her husband. Here blood is invoked in a dramatic bid to refuse patriarchal domestic order. In "Menstruation and Liminality in Ingmar Bergman's *Cries and Whispers*," Ohlin uses the concept of liminality to elaborate the ways in which blood as both form and content—and ritual—defies cinematic narrative (and hence authoritative) coherence.

Kasia van Schaik analyzes Alice Munro's "Juliet" triptych with express emphasis on the short story "Chance." On a train—movement and interrupted movement are in the air—Juliet, a school teacher, contends with her period, which calls for "reinforcements." The "messes"—the irresolution—of a woman's life are the stuff of Munro's short stories, and Van Schaik argues that the female complaint is not just a material thing but a mode—in this case, one whose generic features also suit the form of the short story. In this way, "'The Problem Was That She Was a Girl': The Female Complaint in Alice Munro's Juliet Triptych" shares some of the concerns that Ohlin addresses in his discussion of Bergman and cinema.

Katerina Symes looks at the Netflix series *Orange Is the New Black* to consider how the comedic narrative form, the setting of the show in a woman's prison, and the always-already unruly feminine body conspire to expose and contain at the same time. References to menstrual blood and products are overt, in some instances shocking, humorous, and a source of narrative frustration. Menstrual blood is used to taunt others, and menstrual products are tragically in short supply; they are fought over and repurposed to comedic effect. In "*Orange Is the New Black*: Menstruation, Comedy, and the Unruly Feminine," Symes notes how non-normative scenes of menstrual display fit within the narrative form of comedy and its use of irony—that is, are disciplined by both as well by the constraints of the small screen. This push and pull, the flamboyance, leakiness, and their parodic excess are softened within comedic conventions and are both transgressive and reigned in at the same time.

"Every woman has one," MacDonald says, "a blood story, that is" (340). The chapters in this book amplify menstrual blood so that it performs the various stories it is positioned discursively to do. These stories—there is not just one and that is the point—are, indeed, part of a larger conversation; they inspire dissensus, and open onto liminal spaces that elude precision (and hence partake of the possibilities of unstoppable imagination). Stories about Jacqueline Kennedy Onassis's stories are phantasmatic, given she would not speak publically. Her menstrual blood is her uterine utterance, providing access to her presumably authentic feelings and the faux-intimacy of the fan-celebrity pact. Terry Schiavo's menstrual cycle was a contested site, as it moved from her body to the body of law. The pornographic model foregrounds, in the background, the volatility of blood with a vengeance. Some contemporary ads and marketing for menstrual products are new and welcome interlocutors. Art is a visually semantic conversation. The cinematic plays with reality to resignify what blood can or cannot mean and asks the question of both: what are their symbolic functions? Alice Munro's short stories themselves, and with the menstrual period in particular, accentuate the female complaint itself. And the formal restraints of comedy, the niche context of on demand viewing, conspire to give just enough movement to women who, in the end, while funny and bleeding—two instances of disruptive comportment—are still in prison. But, still: maybe blood is the new black.

Works Cited

"1953 Kotex Ad 'Not a Shadow of a Doubt.'" *Vintage Adventures*, www.vintage-adventures.com/vintage-healthcare-medical-dental-ads/1095-1953-kotex-ad-not-a-shadow-of-a-doubt.html. Accessed 24 Feb. 2019.

"1980 Carefree Panty Shields Ad—Having Fresh Panties." *Vintage Paper Ads*, 2019, www.vintagepaperads.com/1980-Carefree-Panty-Shields-Ad-Having-Fresh-Panties_p_101224.html. Accessed 24 Feb. 2019.

"A Woman's Plight: Learning from Frustration." *History: Preserved*, 28 Dec. 2017, http://www.history-preserved.com/2017/12/a-womans-plight-learning-from.html. Accessed 24 Feb. 2019.

"Because Modess." *Mum*, 1999, http://www.mum.org/modbec.htm. Accessed 24 Feb. 2019.

Bobel, Chris. *New Blood: Third Wave Feminism and the Politics of Menstruation*. Rutgers University Press, 2010.

Butler, Judith. *Bodies That Matter: On the Discursive Limits of Sex*. Routledge, 1993.

"Case Studies." *Andy Tyler*, 2015, https://andytyler.com/projects/5753675. Accessed 24 Feb. 2019.

Fahs, Breanne. *Out For Blood: Essays on Menstruation and Resistance*. SUNY, 2016.

Greer, Germaine. *The Female Eunuch*. Paladin, 1970.

Grosz, Elizabeth. *Volatile Bodies: Toward a Corporeal Feminism*. Indiana University Press, 1994.

"Jack's Story." *Jack Spicer III*, http://www.jackspiceriii.com/new-page. Accessed 24 Feb. 2019.

Kaite, Berkeley. "The Body and Femininity in Feminine Hygiene Advertising." *Culture and Communication: Methodology, Behavior, Artifacts and Institutions*, vol. III, edited by Sari Thomas. Ablex, 1986, pp. 159-167.

Kane, Kate. "The Ideology of Freshness in Feminine Hygiene Commercials." *Journal of Communication Inquiry*, vol. 14, no. 1, 1990, pp. 82-92.

Kissling, Elizabeth Arveda. *Capitalizing on the Curse: The Business of Menstruation.* Lynne Rienner Publishers, 2006.

MacDonald, Shauna M. "Leaky Performances: The Transformative Potential of Menstrual Leaks." *Women's Studies in Communication,* vol. 30, no. 3, fall 2007, pp. 340-357.

Mandziuk, Roseann M. "'Ending Women's Greatest Hygienic Mistake': Modernity and the Mortification of Menstruation in Kotex Advertising, 1921–1926," *Women's Studies Quarterly,* vol. 38, nos. 3-4, fall-winter, 2010, pp. 42-62.

Munro, Alice. "Chance." *Runaway.* McClelland and Stewart, 2004, pp. 48-86.

"New Freedom Feminine Hygiene Magazine Ad Lot * Pads Panty Liners Kotex." *Ebay,* www.ebay.com/itm/NEW-FREEDOM-feminine-hygiene-magazine-ad-lot-pads-panty-liners-Kotex-/ 372315768889? _trksid=p2047675.m43663.144720&nordt= true&rt=nc&orig_cvip=true. Accessed 24 Feb. 2019.

Roach, Joseph. "Culture and Performance in the Circum-Atlantic World." *Performativity and Performance,* edited by Andrew Parker and Eve Kosofsky Sedgwick, Routledge, 1995, pp. 45-63.

Rosewarne, Lauren. *Periods in Pop Culture: Menstruation in Film and Television.* Lexington Books, 2012.

"Sharp Eyes Cannot Tell without Tampax." *Duke University Libraries,* repository.duke.edu/dc/adaccess/BH0169. Accessed 24 Feb. 2019.

"Stay Dry During Downpours." *Slideshare, LinkedIn,* 2010, www.slideshare.net/xamhon/fitness-2010-01. Accessed 24 Feb. 2019.

Steinem, Gloria. *Outrageous Acts and Everyday Rebellions.* New American Library, 1983.

"The Last Enemy To Be Conquered Is Mother Nature: Menstruation in Advertising." *Reed,* 2011 www.reed.edu/anthro/adprojects/2011/case_jacobson_spillane/. Accessed 24 Feb. 2019.

"Why Do Kotex Napkins Protect When Others Fail." *Gogd.tjs Labs,* gogd.tjs-labs.com/show-picture?id=1221758703&size=NORM. Accessed 24 Feb. 2019.

Chapter One

Bloody Jackie: How Menstrual Blood Speaks for Jacqueline Kennedy Onassis's Silence

Berkeley Kaite

Jacqueline Bouvier Kennedy Onassis is famous for a few things, her marriages to President Kennedy and Greek billionaire Aristotle Onassis among them. However, she achieved renown, if not celebrity, from having sat beside JFK in the convertible when he was assassinated. Moreover, there is one image that has come to stand in for her: the bloodied pink suit she was wearing that day in Dallas in November 1963. No mention of the assassination is complete without reference to the pink Chanel suit[1] and its bloody stains. Here is a recent example: "Smeared with her husband's blood and brains ... Her suit and stockings tainted with blood ... her bloody clothes ... The sight of the typically immaculate fashion plate in blood-stained clothes becomes one of the memorable images associated with this tragic weekend" (George 38, 44, 46).

Jackie Kennedy is, indeed, synonymous with blood. Her indelible association with the assassination in Dallas, Texas, is underscored not only by being beside JFK but also by being the recipient of his blood and brains following the final shot that killed him.[2] She is reported to have said, "No, I want them to see what they have done" when beseeched to change out of her suit for the plane ride back to Washington (Manchester 348; Bedell Smith 442; Bradford 274).

Photos of her in the suit with dark bloodstains on her skirt and stockings visually inscribe the assassination on her, and she, even more than her slain husband, is a metonym for the mysteries that attend it: we do not know who killed JFK or why. Two weeks after the assassination *Life* magazine featured Jackie and her children on its cover—a photo of them taken while they wait to follow the president's casket in a cortege to the Capitol building. The accompanying story is "Kennedy's Last Journey," and the editorial of this issue refers to "that bloody weekend" and its several "myths" (not Barthesian myths but rather "the right things to remember") (4). One of the things listed is the "courage and dignity of Jacqueline Kennedy throughout her ordeal" (4). The issue contains a two-page encomium to her with regard to her comportment in the days following the assassination. A year later *Look* magazine put out "The JFK Memorial Issue" (1964). On its cover is not President Kennedy but Jacqueline and John Jr. seated in her lap. The association of Jacqueline Kennedy to the event that ended her husband's life extended into her marriage to Aristotle Onassis, and it followed her to her death and into the present day.[3] *Life* magazine, in an issue commemorating the news events of 1994, the year of Jackie's death, contains a medium close-up of her on its cover, even though that was also the year Richard Nixon died and Nelson Mandela was elected South Africa's first black president (1995). It is notable that her death is offered as the visual moniker of the year, a rather nostalgic and oblique shout-out to an event long past. However, in this photo, which dominates the cover, Jackie is, as always in these retrospectives, in her early thirties and not sixty-four, the age she died. These photos return her to the assassination, that time when she stopped speaking publically. Although the assassination is the implosive event that solidified her celebrity, she would not speak about it after the "Camelot" interview. In that interview with journalist Theodore White, also for *Life* magazine, she notes in grizzly terms what she remembers about JFK when he was shot ("I could see a piece of his skull coming off ... his blood and brains were in my lap... I kept holding the top of his head down trying to keep the brains in") and in which she coin the mythical term "Camelot" to refer to JFK's presidency.[4] Thus, her image, frozen at that time of mystery and silence, fetishizes the spectacularly bloody assassination and all its attendant unknowns. The front cover of *People*'s "The Most Intriguing People of the Century"

(1997) features Jackie Kennedy (among others, for example Martin Luther King Jr., Franklin Roosevelt, and Elizabeth Taylor). Not her first husband, the slain president, but his widow who is described as "treasured for ... charm and sophistication ... as well as the grace and orchestrating intelligence she displayed in the aftermath of the assassination" (52).

Yes, Jacqueline Kennedy Onassis invokes blood and intrigue. So much of her is splayed out and recycled in the media,[5] yet so little of what she knew, thought, or felt is known. Her husband's blood is seared onto both visual and discursive memory of her; indeed, it is a stand-in for her. Therefore, is it a surprise when Edward Klein, in one of the many biographies of her, invokes her menstrual blood? Twenty-five years following the assassination, in *Just Jackie: Her Private Years* (1998), Klein is the first to do so. He introduces the subject of Jackie's menstrual blood in the context of her preparation on the morning of the assassination and sets it up this way: Jack and Jacqueline Kennedy will attend a Chamber of Commerce breakfast in Fort Worth on the morning of 22 November, 1963, before they board Air Force One for the thirteen-minute plane ride to Dallas. Jackie arrives late to this breakfast. This is how Klein tells it[6]: Jack Kennedy, "in a light drizzle," addressed an "outdoor rally of union men" who wanted to know where Jackie was. He told them, "'Mrs. Kennedy is organizing herself. It takes her a little longer, but, of course, she looks better than we do when she does it.'" Klein continues:

> The truth was, Jackie was delayed because she had just begun her menstrual period. It was her first normal monthly flow since Patrick Bouvier had been delivered by cesarean section, and she remembered that it filled her with joy. She and Jack had talked about having more children, but she feared that she might never get pregnant again. So the day that ended in blood had begun in blood, but the first blood was a sign of life. It meant that Jackie could begin to try to have another baby. (9)[7]

Why the need to mention Jackie's menstrual blood, especially amid the shocking and dramatic events that soon followed and for which Jacqueline Kennedy is known? What does her menstrual blood perform in the narrative reconstruction of her life and her death? I argue that although it is a surprising inclusion, it also is not. Jackie's most interior blood is implored to tell a story. The emphasis on Jackie's menstrual blood conflates her vagina with her mouth, her bloody flow with an embodied utterance.

Klein invokes Jackie's menstrual blood to capture a mood of anxious anticipation— Jackie's, JFK's and the crowd's, and now the reader's— and to play with the idea of timing and postponement. However, there is something else at work here—an insistence that deep inside Jackie lie mysteries, a story to tell. All mysteries are metaphorically deep before they are brought to light and no longer mysterious. A self-evident truth is revealed in the comment about Jackie's wish for more children. This much we know: she did not have any more.

Klein's discursive reconstruction of Jackie's early-morning unforeseen contingency before the day's fateful events leads to the excavation of Jackie's body. He discusses her fear that the possible publication of JFK's autopsy reports would expose the president's "chronic venereal disease" (54). From this supposition about JFK's philandering and resultant ill health and of Jackie's feelings about the autopsy, Klein then quotes a doctor who discusses the effects of "nongonococcal urethritis" in a man on his female sexual partner. Klein's aim is to probe more deeply inside his subject—Jackie—and uses his informant to make his case. The doctor concludes, "after the first intercourse, the woman always becomes infected, and the bacteria usually stays [sic] behind and multiplies, and her subsequent pregnancies can be affected. Her second baby might come to term immature, and subsequent pregnancies can be miscarried" (55). From this, Klein himself concludes that Jackie "suffered severe bouts of postpartum depression … and … felt so despondent" following the birth of John Jr. (55), but not before hypothesizing Jackie's interior space by quoting the doctor's abstract assessment—he did not treat either Kennedy—of the effects of venereal disease on a woman's reproductive system. The doctor allows that the bacteria "do not stay inside the woman's uterine canal solely; they go through her tubes, her pelvic cavity, her ovaries, and they interfere with ovarian function. Those sluggish ovaries do not produce the normal complement of hormones" (55). Through the colonization of Jackie's body, Klein himself is anything but "sluggish," as he embellishes all he can to create some metaphoric noise around Jackie's decades-long silent body. If this body could speak, Klein suggests, it would reveal its complex and messy interiors, which, in turn, would verify rumours about JFK's extramarital sexual activity. While indeed the stuff of rumours, conjecture, innuendo, and memoir, these alleged affairs remain even more tantalizing due to their frangibility.[8] Blood here performs the need to know, and the impossibility of it. In invoking JFK's sexual prowess, real or imagined, spilled blood returns to the ethos of the masculine leader, the Byronic figure who "lived like an aristocrat, loved like a libertine, died like a hero" (Lubin 107). David Lubin calls John Kennedy an emblem of the "007 ethos" of the Cold War, combining a roguish "confirmation of potency, sexual or otherwise" with the "Romantic ideology of derring-do" (109). Neither Jack's body nor his will is sluggish: rather, both are the stuff of the vigorous rake (Lubin 44).

Jack was not lethargic, but Jackie's ovaries are assumed to be. They and her fallopian tubes are presented as the royal route to the enduring secrets of the assassination, to be sure, but also to what preceded it and what the assassination really eliminated: insider knowledge of the celebrities JFK and Jackie themselves.[9] Jackie's "pelvic cavity" (empty indeed) is the foil for her empty mouth, the mouth that would not speak (more on this below).

As Klein says: "There was blood everywhere. Not only on Jackie's hair and gloves and skirt and stockings. Her panties were soaked with menstrual blood, too. She was covered in blood from head to foot ... She felt that if she let go of Jack, she would collapse in their commingled blood" (10).

Jack and Jackie's blood is "commingled" in many ways. It is literally so, but we are only talking about Jacqueline Kennedy because Jack's story bleeds into hers (and vice versa). *America's Queen: The Life of Jacqueline Kennedy Onassis* (2000) by Sarah Bradford begins with praise for Jackie's performance at JFK's funeral. Bradford calls her introduction "Four Days in America: November 22-25, 1963"; she leads with a quote from an American ambassador and assistant to Attorney General Robert F. Kennedy who notes how Jackie "became indelibly inscribed on the mind of anyone who watched the event. All of her life, I think, people who had seen that, and those days, never thought of her any other way" (ix). Jackie is memorialized in this way, forever an emblem for "Camelot"—a version of her husband's presidency, itself retroactively connoting a "court" (Bedell Smith xi-xv)—whose invocation was only inaugurated following his death.

Bradford employs mythical figures to invoke Jackie's status as an "icon, a legend beyond the scope of ordinary experience" (ix). It is JFK's mode of death that secures a retelling of the funeral featuring Jackie as "marble ... an ancient statue... as if she represented all the heroes' widows down the centuries since Andromache mourned Hector outside the walls of Troy ... she created a myth" (Bradford ix). Indeed, few would remember, write, or talk about Jacqueline Kennedy Onassis, in the way they do, if not for her spectacular association with her husband's spectacular death.[10]

The blood of the martyred leader may overdetermine Jackie's blood, but her blood is still charged with a performance of its own. Blood is after all extracted from this "marble ... statue ... myth." Reference to her menstrual blood opens onto a story untold, although there is no real story; therefore, whether real or not, Klein imagines it. Jan Pottker later picks it up in *Janet and Jackie: The Story of a Mother and Her Daughter, Jacqueline Kennedy Onassis* (2001). She writes that in Fort Worth, early on the morning of 22 November, 1963, Jackie is keeping the president, and "two thousand excited Texans in attendance" waiting (213). Her menstrual blood is worked into a narrative of anticipatory excitement: Jackie is "still irritated" with her personal secretary; she is "running behind schedule, which did not improve her mood." Jack instructs an aide to find out what is keeping Jackie; he tells the crowd, which "roared in appreciation," that she is "organizing herself"; and then Jackie "descend[s] with her Secret Service agents ... twenty minutes late" (212-13). She is behind schedule because she "had awakened and found that she was menstruating, so it took her a little longer to get ready" (212). The discovery of menstrual blood, normally a prosaic event, is here presented as narrative punctuation: it structures the story in the telling of it. If it were its own punctuation mark, it would be a colon, for it announces that something is coming, is about to happen, is itself about to be "awakened and found" (though only in retrospect and only in the way we care about the assassination, given it needs to be rewritten in the hope of achieving narrative closure).

When Pottker picks up the anecdote, she uses it, as does Klein, to summon retroactively dramatic tension leading up to the assassination. Jackie's discovery of her menstrual blood is an event that will culminate in an exploding head—captured on the home video of Abraham Zapruder—and these narrated details underscore the inevitability of that histrionic death. But, still: why is menstrual blood in the air? It both delays the big event and it presages it. It tells a bloody story in a story whose motif is blood. But it also imputes guilt by association to Jackie herself. She will be covered in blood, very soon, and what will she have to say about that? Nothing. It must be stressed that this reference to her menstrual blood comes decades after the assassination, decades filled with fruitless excavation of the various conspiracy theories and scrutiny of every possible angle related to the assass-ination, JFK's alleged assassin Lee Harvey Oswald, Jack Ruby, the man who murdered Oswald, etc. The Kennedys are a "cultural screen saver: not a day goes by without our seeing their images" (Mallon 171). It is as if her/his/our discovery of the blood will finally reveal what we have been waiting to hear: what was going on inside Jackie, the person closest to the president when the bullets struck? The introduction to the hardback edition of a compilation of witness testimonies to the Warren Commission (released in 1964 and investigated the assassination) opens with a quote from Jackie's testimony—"All I remember is seeing my husband, he had this quizzical look on his face"(vii)—but her post-assassination demeanour betrays nothing. The paperback version contains photos on both inside flaps; the caption accompanying Jacqueline's refers to her as a "witness" to the assassination. The latent question is what can she produce? What will she offer up freely, spontaneously, authentically, truthfully, and without guile? In these reimaginings her blood is seen as her unwilled, even if desired, (uterine) utterance. Klein sees it as wishful—promising a future conception, a baby and, you can read between the lines, a repeat male heir—yet it is his/our desire to colonize the body that now stands in for the president's slain body and the unsolved mysteries around it. Jackie did witness JFK's head shattered by the bullet, but the Zapruder footage makes clear she is looking at him, not outside the car or at anyone else: she is not a witness who can provide any answers. Even if she could have, she would not and would remain closed lipped in the face of a public beseeching her to speak about the assassination.

Pottker does not subject Jackie to a gynecological assessment but writes that on Air Force One, while waiting for the plane to return to Washington with JFK's body, Jackie "continued to sit, alone with her thoughts. She later said, 'in Dallas they gave me red roses, I thought how funny – red roses – so all the seat was full of blood and red roses'

... She used the bathroom and noticed, again, that she had her period. She wept once more—Patrick gone, Jack gone—red blood and red roses. She returned to the bedroom and sat alone with her thoughts" (221). In the cultural imaginary Jackie is not alone with her thoughts for very long, as those thoughts are conceived and dreamt of, written and rewritten, and ventriloquized by a nation of voyeur-biographers. However, it is assumed her thoughts are there, that she is preoccupied by them— understandably so—and that she must be prized open in order that we may be privy to them. Jackie's menstrual blood is an epitaph of her (our) thoughts: past, present and future. *Past*: what did she know about JFK's rumoured affairs and what was the state of their marriage? Did she love him? Did his alleged venereal diseases cause Jackie's miscarriage in 1954? Nevertheless, assumed ruminations of her personal past are also a foil for what she might have seen and might have known of the assassination. Yet, what Jackie knew and saw—what anyone knew or saw— remains elusive and, thus, is the enduring epistemological wound.

And there are the demonstratively *present* thoughts: all talk of Jacqueline Bouvier Kennedy Onassis, even during and following the Onassis chapter of her life, fastens onto the assassination: its attendant details are routinely, freshly embellished to enliven the historical record. In *Jacqueline Bouvier Kennedy Onassis: The Untold Story* (2014), Barbara Leaming writes during the months following the assassination that Jackie "rehearsed the same brief sequence" (126) (i.e., what happened in the motorcade) and she returns to a self-lacerating comment Jackie offered in her brief testimony to the Warren Commission. Leaming writes, "If only she had been looking to the right, she told herself, she might have saved her husband. If only she had recognized the sound of the first shot, she could have pulled him down in time" (126). The repressed returns never to let the past recede; it enacts the past in the present and holds it in melancholic reverie. Therefore, Jackie's private ruminations prefigure a *future*:—menstrual-themed thoughts, so to speak—about what might have happened, point to the potential of unborn children and what that could have said about JFK's and Jackie's marriage. Klein has Jackie's menstrual blood performing a future of unknowns yet, with hindsight, sluggish with impossibilities. If Jackie had the thoughts he attributes to her, if she wanted more children even after the still-born baby, the miscarriage and now the death of Patrick at two days old, her abstract desires are set in motion, yet unspoken and unrealized. And given that Klein's suppositions are in a biography written a few years after Jackie's death, the presumed longing for more children, we now know, was a thwarted one, for Jackie never had another child. Her menstrual blood in this telling of the future is replete with (fantasized) yearning and its frustration (yearning and its frustration being a good definition of desire). However, this sort of imagining of the future keeps desire in motion, and this includes perhaps foremost the desires of the cultural ventriloquist—the fan—for mastery of the story. Klein fills out Jackie's story by filling in the blanks, in this case rather literally, her blank insides, her "cavity," a masquerade for the cavity left by the mysteries around the assassination of JFK. Inside, Jackie is both life and death, excess and silence—the future but with nothing imminent save for the fecund field of biographers and historians who can control the narrative, even if it relies on the relentless fantasization of what might have been. In fact, the unknowns themselves are desirable, as they propel a narcissistic drive to see oneself in the image of one's own creation (Reynolds).

Jackie holds things up and later struggles to hold things in. She is the frustrating figure of containment that her menstrual blood, in turn, frustrates. I want to argue here that Jackie's most significant orifice is not her vagina—from which her menstrual blood issued—but, in fact, her mouth. Jackie was strategically silent following the assassination; she refused to speak beyond a few empty phrases of her reactions to the vivid and shocking murder of her husband. She would not speak casually to reporters; she did not give interviews (beyond the "Camelot" interview with Theodore White in 1981, which she was allowed to edit), nor would she partake of the autobiography craze. She would not appear on talk shows, and she successfully sued paparazzo photographer Ron Galella for intruding into her private life ("One Man's"). When anyone deigned to reveal what she considered too much, she either initiated the threat of lawsuits (Manchester) or excised them from her life (Bradlee). And perhaps the most gossipy element in her life, if still only the forceful and enduring stuff of rumour—her husband's infidelities—is a subject she would not touch.[11] Jackie would not speak.

Jackie would not speak, so when she died, there were more

biographies of her than any other living American woman (Thomas 34). A nation of ventriloquists stepped in to imagine and fill the silence—a silence all the more remarkable given the many uncertainties that inform the assassination—built into the lives and relationships of Jack and Jackie Kennedy during and after the presidency. Jackie's mouth is yet another metonym for JFK's death and all the secrets both of them took to their graves.

Her mouth produced nothing; the biographer, though, has her vagina flowing profusely. I argue Jackie's menstrual blood performs the need to have her speak and gestures to all that she may spontaneously and effortlessly divulge. Blood is her body's confession and a foil for her absent speech. Menstrual blood is the body's admission, its "plethora" (Laqueur 35). Thomas Laqueur resurrects "plethora" from early Hippocratic accounts to invoke primitive, but apparently persistent and durable, associations between the womb and the neck (35-36). He uses the word in its original sense to note helpfully its reference to an excess of blood in the circulation system.

Here are Laqueur's observations: ancient wisdom had it that menstrual blood was a "plethora or leftover of nutrition ... in this generic economy of fluids and organs" (35). It was understood that the breastfeeding mother converted surplus blood into milk and, thus, did not menstruate. Thus, the "normal plethora" transformed into other embodiments: fat in the obese, movement in dancers, and vocal expression in singers (36). The assumption that menstrual blood was excessive and transferrable is of interest, as it underscores the notion of the volatility of blood, its mutability and unpredictability; blood is never only one thing. This connection between excess blood and the throat and voice appears, in the case of Jackie Kennedy at least, to linger in the popular imaginary. However, one has to add not just with this iconic figure. In the 2016 American presidential campaign, Republican candidate, and now president, Donald Trump later remarked about moderator Megyn Kelly's pointed questions regarding his comments on women during a televised debate on Fox News: "you could see there was blood coming out of her eyes, blood coming out of her wherever."[12] Here the imagined blood is summoned to represent Kelly's will, intellect, and presence on the stage—she is simply doing her job—as well as Trump's inability to control her words, and it is a foil for Trump's own anger: Kelly's phantom blood returns to attack

Trump in two ways. The first is in the form of her rhetoric. In her questions, Kelly, in fact, quotes Trump back to himself: she asks about his characterizations of women as "fat pigs, dogs, slobs, and disgusting animals." So when he hears his own words spoken by a woman (perhaps in his eyes one of the above slurs), he sees red all over again. Blood and verbal rage, his and then mirrored via Kelly's quotations, are synonymous. Blood and language—the throat and mouth—are twinned. The second form through which the candidate feels under siege is through a variation on the *vagina dentate*: here, the plethora of blood that Trump summons escapes through Kelly's vagina, her "wherever." Not only does "wherever" suggests something difficult or impossible to locate, it also invokes its adjacent compound adverb "everywhere." "Wherever" summons the mythically evasive and elusive feminine; "everywhere" suggests leakiness and what threatens to escape discursive control. Both at once suppress and beckon menstrual blood with their co-dependent assumptions of a threatening presence.

The blood from Kelly's "wherever" is prompted by her speech—her mouth here is contiguous with her vagina and forceful words are equated with spectral menstrual blood—and is assumed to be propelled by its own ability to flow unimpeded. The belief in "fungible" fluids and the "generic corporal economy" (Laqueur 35) endures here in its repressed forms. Laqueur notes the ancient belief that "singers are less likely to menstruate"; their plethora is rerouted to their throats and mouths (36). That is to say, the latent belief is Kelly's plethora of words is best connoted and replaced by menstrual blood in the economy of this man's patriarchal desire. With respect to Jackie, the larger and veiled cultural desire is to hear her story—her voice is fetishized in this[13]—and the words she hoards and conceals are assumed to be betrayed by her bloody utterance.

Note that Klein has Jackie's menstrual blood "soaking" through her "panties" while in the car. This is his embellishment, as his notes indicate that Jackie's mother revealed in an interview only that she discovered her period that morning. Klein's fantasy extends the metaphor of blood to encompass both the leaky—unruly—feminine and the feminine stain.

The Hoover Dam could not stop the flow of words created on Jackie's behalf. The will to get her to speak is as grand as Trump's was to reroute Megyn Kelly's flow of words. Therefore, along with the dozens of biographies of and articles on Jacqueline Kennedy Onassis, Klein excavates Jackie Kennedy's interior space[14] and then fills it with an unrelenting flow of blood. She's drenched in blood, JFK's and now her own from within. She is written in blood—just as JFK's deathly blood underwrites her place in history—and hers is of the uncontrollable kind: the return of her menstrual period after the birth and early death of Patrick were unexpected. The assumption is she was caught unawares and so needed extra time, but for what? Klein speculates that the return of Jackie's period meant she could get pregnant again, and this is what she wanted. Jackie's plethora promises to furnish the future. But this is Klein's fantasy; moreover, it does not come to fruition. The menstrual blood fuses with the deathly blood; it is only invoked because of the latter and is inscribed in the years following the assassination in a dramatic bid to fill in the enduring silence. Both the menstrual blood and JFK's blood are stains that represent the unspoken and the unspeakable.

Jackie's bloody mess defiled her clothes and JFK's bloody demise did as well. But there is more abstract defilement at work and that returns to the fan's peculiar need to see the celebrity knocked down, metaphorically bloodied, stained, tarred and caught unawares in unscripted moments. Not for nothing, a TV announcer declares shortly after the assassination was reported that Jackie "is heard to have uttered 'Oh, no,'" such a mundane yet somehow noteworthy proclamation (*JFK: 3 Shots That Changed America*). The unscripted verbal and uterine utterance fascinates and marks the occasion. Blood, words, silence, and mysterious insides all co-mingle here.

Any speculation of Jackie Kennedy has to be a spotty reconstruction based on what was written about her and the very little she let out in restrained form. She was an educated woman, shy, often awkward in front of the TV camera and microphone. Her charisma comes in part from her still photographs—she was indeed photogenic—but also her enduring reserve as well as her ability to contain, refuse, and defer. Her silence defers the story and keeps it going. ("Blood Stains Tell Tale" is the *Chicago Tribune* caption that accompanies a photo of Jackie in her pink suit upon arriving in Washington from Texas [Hutchinson 1]) It does seem clear that she wanted to craft carefully her public image and to control the media's access to her children. The reticence for which she is known follows her already-established celebrity presence—a status that was cinched for having witnessed the assassination with the physical and emotional proximity of none other. Yet she would not confess to what she saw, knew, or felt. It is left to others to fill in that story-in-waiting. Blood by contrast is noisy, loud, colourful, and, more to the point, uncontrollable.

To conclude, I offer a few words on the defiled celebrity. One cannot talk about Jacqueline Kennedy without invoking the words glamour and celebrity. "America's Newest Star!" shouted the October 1961 cover of *Photoplay*. Neither glamour nor celebrity is a self-evident concept; both in fact are rather spongy and absorb a lot. It is their lack of clear definition that renders them malleable, slippery, and mythical in the sense that they affirm ideological values so embedded in cultural life as to seem "natural" (Barthes). I bring these up, as I want to argue they intersect in significant ways with the insinuation of blood into Jacqueline Kennedy Onassis. JFK's blood and Jackie's own menstrual blood are, again and as with all blood, not singular in their meaning. Her menstrual blood is invoked to tell a story—that cannot be told— and to tarnish Jackie's glamour and her celebrity presence. How does this work? In his book *Glamour: A History* (2008), Stephen Gundle usefully notes that glamour derives from the "culture of the bourgeois era ... of image-making, of masks and appearances" (10) and the culture of the theatre, the "world of representation, where play-acting and fakery were commonplace" (10). Glamour is, thus, intrinsically about the orchestration of the surface and the marketing of its image. Gundle notes of Jackie Kennedy that her particular allure was the result of the "borrowed auras" from screen stars (304). She was, indeed, featured in the same movie magazines as Elizabeth Taylor, and even if they were seen as contrasts, they occupied the same cultural space. The cover of *Photoplay*, June 1962, reads "America's 2 Queens! Jacqueline Kennedy vs. Elizabeth Taylor: A comparison of their days and nights! How they raise their children! How they treat their men!" Both these women are glamorous, yet each in her own way. Gundle argues that glamour—a slippery concept so hard to define—contains its own binary, one-half of which is tantalizing, enthralling, and "instantly perceptible" (2ff). The other half, with its roots in theatricality, is characterized by simulation. Wayne Koestenbaum reinforces this idea when he refers to Jackie and Liz as each having a *soupçon* of "vulgarity ... Jackie was pseudo-French; Liz was pseudo-British" (72). Glamour is part artifice and, therefore, averse to authenticity. Jackie's menstrual blood can be seen in this instance as the uncensored picture of truthfulness. Glamour is adjacent to, and overlaps with, the tarnished image.

The celebrity image is also one we wish to see defiled. A psycho-analytic interpretation of this manoeuvre centres on the fan's need to shame the star. We could say that, like blood, the celebrity is in a liminal and fluid state. She occupies the whimsy, desires, and *schadenfreude* of the fan. Richard Schickel calls this the "envious psychodrama" of adoration and punishment that attends to the fan-celebrity relationship (169). To bloody Jackie metaphorically—for this is what happens each time mention is made of the suit covered with JFK's blood, brains, and gore—is to partake in the phenomenon of celebrity defilement. This is a noisy slip of the collective tongue: photos in the gossip-pages frame the desire to catch the celebrity unawares in unscripted moments, especially those in which the star trips up and tries to avoid the camera, and frequently contain the vernacular "resting bitch face." These moments are perceived to be authentic and true, and to reveal the real person behind the façade. But they are also aimed to shame the celebrity. Part of the unconscious machinations of the celebrity-fan pact is the fan's need for recognition from the mirror or screen that is the star's image. However, the star will not return that gaze and note here the proliferation of photographs in which Jackie wears sunglasses—her refusal to speak is visually reinforced.[15] This is the "fame damage" (Redmond 34) to which fans are attached and seek out: the downfalls and slip-ups of the star that result in the real or metaphoric wounded body (Johansson 352). As Jacqueline Rose puts it, "celebrity is often a ritual of public humiliation" (10); spectators' shame at the shallow indulgence in the lives of others. Rose argues the embarrassment that accompanies the deep engagement in the lives of strangers—whose experiences are so far removed from our own and so often accompanied by dismissal and denial—is projected onto the celebrities drawn of our cannibalistic hunger. That is, the celebrity presence points to the co-mingling of apparent binary opposites of pleasure and aggression, reverence and (symbolic) defilement. Celebrities are our guilty and public secrets—ciphers for our more forbidden impulses and the repository for things we wish to keep repressed yet, for which we seek an outlet. The need to revere and the need to humiliate are co-habitants of the celebrity-fan unspoken agreement. And that pact underlies the assassination of JFK and the way it itself released unspeakable aggression wrapped up in an oedipal drama writ large. In "The Glassy Knoll: Identity, Identification, and Desire in Kennedy Narratives," Mike Reynolds writes of "the curiously pliable Kennedy clay," (86) the representative character necessary for America's "'romantic dream of itself'" (Mailer qtd. in Reynolds 83). If "we need identity not to be there, so that we can really find it" (Reynolds 86) then that figure needs to be out of the way so we can fill in the gaps with our own ferocious desires: desire needs absence so that it can be kept in play. The unspeakable, thus, is the unconscious desire for the spectacular demise of JFK. Jackie's silence following the gaps and absences around the assassination—who did it and why—becomes another gap and absence. Co-joined with her celebrity presence, blood as punishment speaks to the scene of a couple of crimes. One is the crime of the assassination, and another is the necessary defacement accompanying star status.

Menstrual blood is performative, and Jackie's noted glamour does not contradict the desire to showcase her blood; rather it is what secures it. It is the glamourous star image that is in need of disciplining, and that discipline takes the form of a seeping stain. The leakiness of Jackie's blood appears to violate the celebrity-fan contract, but it, in fact, reveals it for what it is: the (unconsciously) logical outcome to the infringement of the fan-celebrity pact. In Jackie's case, this is her silence—her refusal to return the fan's narcissistic gaze and give it what it wants to hear. Blood speaks but never in just one voice.

Endnotes

1. That the suit's provenance cannot be ascertained (i.e., is it an original Chanel, a copy, or a Schiaparelli?), is part of its enduring resonance. Much like its owner and the blood she sported, the suit remains a mystery and is part of the epistemological uncertainty that characterizes the assassination and its aftermath.

2. To recap the events surrounding the assassination: JFK was killed by a bullet to the head while in a convertible in a motorcade in Dallas, Texas, in November 1963. His alleged assassin, Lee Harvey

Oswald, was killed two days later by Jack Ruby; this was caught on live television. An inquiry into these events, the *Report of the President's Commission* (the "Warren Commission"), completed its work in less than a year and concluded that Oswald had acted alone and was not part of a conspiracy to kill the president.

3. Taraborrelli: "There was Jackie, standing alone, in her pink wool suit covered with ugly splotches of dried blood ... there was blood streaked on her cheek" (197-98).

4. One week after the assassination, Jacqueline Kennedy approached journalist Theodore White saying "there was something that she wanted *Life* magazine to say to the country, and I must do it... she wanted me to make certain that Jack was not forgotten in history... I should make clear to the people how much magic there had been in John. F. Kennedy's time. But ... magic is so difficult to capture in any conversation." White wrote up the interview as a two-page insert in the 6 December, 1963, issue of *Life* magazine. It is in the piece that Jackie first coins the term "Camelot" to refer to JFK's presidency. White quotes from the interview: "History! ... It's what those bitter old men write.... Do you know what I think of history? ... When something is written down, does that make it history? The things they say! ... for Jack history was full of heroes" (qtd. in White 523). Claiming that the president would listen to the song from the Broadway musical *Camelot,* Jackie quoted the line "Don't let it be forgot, that once there was a spot, for one brief and shining moment that was known as Camelot." For an account of this meeting, see Theodore H. White. Jackie spoke with William Manchester for *The Death of a President*, but portions of that interview, which do not appear in the book, are under embargo until 2064.

5. As of this writing there is a new biography, see Taraborelli

6. Klein reports that the person who interviewed Jackie's mother for the Kennedy Library's Oral History (371) told him what took place in Jackie's hotel room in Fort Worth the morning of 22 November 1963.

7. Patrick Bouvier Kennedy, who would have been the Kennedy's third child, was born prematurely in August 1963 and lived less than two days.

8. In *Once Upon a Secret: My Affair with President John F. Kennedy and Its Aftermath* (2012), Mimi Alford notes that she destroyed all three pieces of material evidence that she shared an intimate relationship with the president. She claims she wanted to honour her promise to him that she would not reveal their affair. Mary Pinchot Meyer is also rumoured to have had a sexual relationship with JFK, yet her diary, in which she writes of the affair, was destroyed. See Burleigh and Bradlee.

9. Also, this puts an end to JFK as the source of political intrigue of the time—his feelings about Cuba, the Bay of Pigs, etc.

10. Some have written about Jacqueline Kennedy under the rubric of "first ladies" studies (Caroli; Gould; Means). What concerns me here is the iconographic rendition of Jacqueline Kennedy Onassis, the ways in which she is inscribed as part of the cultural imaginary.

11. On the occasion of the release of interviews between Jacqueline Kennedy and Arthur M. Schlesinger, Jr., recorded in 1964, ABC news did a small story on this, and Diane Sawyer asked Caroline Kennedy if her mother ever spoke about her marriage with her, Caroline demurred on this saying, "I wouldn't be her daughter if I answered that" ("Jacqueline Kennedy In Her Own Words").

12. This was uttered on CNN on 7 August 2015, following the 6 August debate on Fox News.

13. Many comment on her voice. White, for example, refers to the "particular whispering intimacy of Jacqueline Kennedy's voice" (522).

14. Klein includes an anecdote of Jackie having lunch with a friend shortly before she died. Normally, "Jackie would never touch" dessert, but this day, she "plowed through" five of them (365-66). It's an odd thing to include about a person's last days, but it goes to reimagining Jackie's interior space and to filling it up.

15. An obituary note indicates the ways in which she conspired against the fan's need for narcissistic recognition: "she seemed like someone who could take us or leave us ... she didn't seem to need us ... she was a mystery ... she was not interested in having a relationship with us" (Johnson 148).

Works Cited

Alford, Mimi. *Once Upon a Secret: My Affair with President John F. Kennedy and Its Aftermath.* Random House, 2012.

Barthes, Roland. 1957. *Mythologies.* Translated by Annette Lavers. Farrar, Straus and Giroux, 1972.

Bedell-Smith. *Grace and Power: The Private World of the Kennedy White House.* Random House, 2004.

Bradford, Sarah. *America's Queen: The Life of Jacqueline Kennedy Onassis.* Viking, 2000.

Bradlee, Ben. *A Good Life.* Simon and Schuster, 1995.

Burleigh, Nina. *A Very Private Woman: The Life and Unsolved Murder of Presidential Mistress Mary Meyer.* Bantam, 1998.

Caroli, Betty Boyd. *First Ladies.* Oxford, 1995.

George, Alice L. *The Assassination of John F. Kennedy: Political Trauma and American Memory.* Routledge, 2013.

Gould, Lewis L. *American First Ladies: Their Lives and Their Legacy.* Taylor and Francis, 2001.

Gundle, Stephen. *Glamour: A History.* Oxford University Press, 2008.

Hutchinson, Louise. "Blood Stains Tell Tale." *Chicago Tribune,* November 23, 1963, p. 1.

"Jacqueline Kennedy In Her Own Words," *YouTube,* 13 Sep. 2011, www.youtube.com/watch?v=ubtlRMTViHA. Accessed 3 Mar. 2019.

"The JFK Memorial Issue," *Look,* November 17, 1964.

JFK: 3 Shots that Changed America. Directed by Nicole Rittenmeyer and Seth Skundrick, The History Channel, 2009.

Johansson, Sofia. "Sometimes You Wanna Hate Celebrities: Tabloid Readers and Celebrity Coverage," *Framing Celebrity: New Directions in Celebrity Culture,* edited by Su Holmes and Sean Redmond, Routledge, 2006, pp. 343-361.

Johnson, Marilyn. "Her Own Woman: An Appreciation of Jacqueline Bouvier Kennedy Onassis." *Life,* July 1994, pp. 48-49.

Klein, Edward. *Just Jackie: Her Private Years.* Ballantine, 1998.

Koestenbaum, Wayne. *Jackie under My Skin: Interpreting an Icon.* Picador, 1995.

Laqueur, Thomas. *Making Sex: Body and Gender from the Greeks to Freud.* Harvard University Press, 1990.

Leaming, Barbara. *Jacqueline Bouvier Kennedy Onassis: The Untold Story.* Thomas Dunne Books, 2014.

Lubin, David M. *Shooting Kennedy: JFK and the Culture of Images.* University of California Press, 2003.

Mallon, Thomas. *Mrs. Paine's Garage and the Murder of John F. Kennedy.* Pantheon, 2002.

Manchester, William. *The Death of a President: November 20-November 25, 1963.* Harper & Row, 1967.

Manchester, William. *Controversy and Other Essays in Journalism, 1950-1975.* Little, Brown & Co., 1980.

Means, Marianne. *The Woman in the White House: The Lives, Times and Influence of Twelve Notable First Ladies.* Random House, 1963.

"One Man's Running Battle with Jackie." *Life,* 31 Mar. 1972.

Pottker, Jan. *Janet and Jackie: The Story of a Mother and Her Daughter, Jacqueline Kennedy Onassis.* St. Martin's Press, 2001.

Redmond, Sean. "Intimate Fame Everywhere." *Framing Celebrity: New Directions in Celebrity Culture,* edited by Su Holmes and Sean Redmond, Routledge, 2006, pp. 27-43.

Report of the President's Commission on the Assassination of President John F. Kennedy. United States Government Publishing Office, 1964.

Reynolds, Mike. "The Glassy Knoll: Identity, Identification, and Desire in Kennedy Narratives," *Journal for the Psychoanalysis of Culture & Society,* vol. 6, no. 1, Spring 2001, pp. 83-96.

Rose, Jacqueline. "The Cult of Celebrity," *London Review of Books, vol. 20, no. 16, 1998, pp. 10-13.*

Schickel, Richard. *Intimate Strangers: The Culture of Celebrity.* Doubleday & Company, Inc., 1985.

Smith, Sally Bedell. *Grace and Power: The Private World of the Kennedy White House.* Random House, 2004.

"Special Collector's Edition," *People,* 1997.

Taraborrelli, J. Randy. *Jackie, Janet & Lee.* St. Martin's, 2018.

Thomas, Evan. "Grace and Iron." *Newsweek,* May 30, 1994, p. 34.

White, Theodore H. *In Search of History: A Personal Adventure*. Warner Books, 1981.

"The 72 Hours and What They Can Teach Us." Editorial, *Life*, 6 Dec., 1963, p. 4.

Chapter Two

"Who Is That 'She'?": Narratives of Menstruation in the Terri Schiavo Case

Claire Horn

We heard about a "she." She, Terri, has her menstrual period. She, Terri, does this or does that. Who is that "she"? If the doctors' diagnoses are correct, which I believe they are, there is no "she" that knows she's having a menstrual period—*In re the Guardianship of Theresa Marie Schiavo,* 975

In the early 2000s, Terri Schiavo—a forty-one-year-old Florida woman who had been in a persistent vegetative state for nearly fifteen years after her unexpected collapse at the age of twenty-six—was at the centre of international attention. The Supreme Court heard evidence from her husband, Michael Schiavo, who requested that his wife's life support be removed, who argued that she would not have wanted to be sustained by artificial measures, and from Terri Schiavo's parents, Robert and Mary Schindler, who believed that their daughter was severely disabled but not beyond recovery.

When a vegetative patient has not left a written will and conflict ensues over that patient's best interests, the court is tasked with trying to construct the patient's preferences by interpreting comments or emotions they expressed in the past, and their beliefs, values, and personality as described by those who knew them. In this unique situation at the intersection of medicine and law, others construct vegetative patients as subjects through the stories told about them. Bioethicists and legal theorists—such as Karla Holloway, Allison August and Steven Miles, Robin Fiore, and Diane Raymond—have examined the differential construction of male and female patients in such cases. These studies demonstrate that gender has an impact on everything from the likelihood that a right to die case will go to court to the chances that the court will accept testimony as to the patient's preferences. August and Miles, in particular, have conducted extensive qualitative studies in which they found that although courts accepted constructions of male patients' wishes based on a range of evidence— "from specific discussions, to general discussions remote from the time and possibility of illness to constructions simply based on the man's character" (89)—the same courts only accepted the construction of women's wishes due to "very specific remarks [about medical treatment]" (89). Medical professionals are less likely to raise concerns over the end of life treatment of male patients, and as August and Miles's findings suggest, "gender profoundly affects judicial analysis of right-to-die cases" (91).

There are a number of narratives that emerged within the Schiavo case that can be traced and analyzed to consider the gendered dimensions of how she was inscribed as a subject. I am interested in a particular element that became a key point of discussion in her case but has received little critical attention—the way in which Schiavo's continued menstruation was read and interpreted in court. Analysis of the differential accounts built around male and female patients in right to die cases is significant beyond simply understanding the assumptions projected onto gendered bodies in the courtroom. These cases sit at the nexus of two of the most powerful institutions in America: the court and the medical system. More importantly, as cases that hold silent bodies waiting to be read and interpreted as their central figures, in which characterizations are presented and judged on their perceived accuracy, these cases are an important site for tracing which kinds of stories and assumptions about male and female subjects are accepted as valid and which are dismissed.

In the Schiavo case, menstrual blood was mobilized as a tool in creating convincing narratives by both legal teams. In a courtroom, the primary duty of a complainant's team is this act of narration: planning the most desirable arc of the trial, prepping witnesses and clients for the kinds of stories they must tell in service of this end, and guiding cross-examination to highlight evidence supporting their discursive constructions.

Schiavo's menstruation is deployed in three ways. Both Michael Schiavo's team, led by George Felos, as well as the Schindler team, led by Pam Campbell, solicited evidence from complainants and witnesses (including Schiavo's family, friends, and physicians) regarding Schiavo's menstruation. George Felos's team used the evidence heard about Schiavo's menstruation to support a narrative in which he framed the excessive nature of Schiavo's menstrual blood as evidence, beyond any other medical complications, that Schiavo was beyond help and her continued care placed an undue burden on those around her. For Felos, Schiavo's heavy menstrual blood represents Schiavo as a woman whose body must be understood as inevitably problematic for both her and others and as a woman who should, therefore, be removed from life support.

Campbell's team, by contrast, used the evidence heard about Schiavo's period to argue that though Schiavo had been vegetative for nearly fifteen years and showed no evidence of cognition, her menstruation demonstrated that she was "just like any other woman" (*Schiavo* 295), and for this reason, she should be sustained on life support. In this rendering, Schiavo is constructed before the court as a generic "woman," who despite her vegetative condition has a body that continues to perform the automatic functions associated with womanhood and is, therefore, perfectly functional. Campbell's team ultimately offers a second, overarching narrative around Schiavo's menstruation in framing Schiavo as a woman who could potentially become a mother and, therefore, should not be allowed to die. Here, menstruation is straightforwardly linked to the desire for motherhood. Both Campbell and Felos wove evidence about Schiavo's menstruation into discussions of whether she had wanted to have children prior to becoming vegetative and whether her continued menstruation meant she could become pregnant. This argumentative thread (which given that Schiavo was vegetative and could never consent to becoming pregnant has disturbing undertones of rape) established Schiavo as a subject that should be read more in relation to her potential efficacy as a mother than as an individual who might have had feelings and opinions about her continued medical treatment.

It is not possible to extrapolate definitively all the discourses of menstruation in broader society from individual delineations emerging in one court case. However, as I have noted above, courts hold significance as sites of subject construction. In order for lawyers and advocates to tell stories in court, they must first gather and certify evidence. The validity of this evidence can be proved or undermined when presented in the court by the opposing legal team's objection and by the judge's discretion to allow or dismiss a line of questioning.

Given the rigor required of lawyers to support their claims, then, the evidence used to construct the scenarios surrounding Schiavo's blood had been assessed on multiple levels (by lawyers on each side of the case, and by the judge) and was found to be acceptable prior to arriving in the courtroom. The contrasting interpretations of Schiavo's period gesture to two social suppositions about menstrual blood in North America: that excessive blood suggests a woman is damaged beyond repair and that regular bleeding is evidence a woman has the utility and aspiration to be a mother.

In the text of the Schiavo trial, Pam Campbell, the Schindlers' lead counsel, keenly cross-examines several witnesses about Schiavo's menstruation. Campbell guides Schiavo's former co-worker, her mother, her sister, and her treating physician to provide evidence about Schiavo's period. In cross-examining Schiavo's mother, Campbell asks, "Did you know that she [Terri] was going to a gynecologist?" (*Schiavo* 347) Her mother replies, "I knew she was, because Terri has always had problems with her period" (347). Later, Campbell questions one of Schiavo's former co-workers about her gynecology appointments. The co-worker, Jackie Rhodes, testifies, "I have a doctor's appointment, and usually mine was like right around there. I know she was having problems with her period" (805). These pieces of evidence—each of which would have been presented to and approved by both the trial judge and Michael Schiavo's legal team prior to being raised in the courtroom—appear to be irrelevant to the question at hand: whether or not Terri Schiavo would want to be sustained on life support. The above discussions, which speak to Shiavo's menstrual habits but not to her preferences for life or death in an end of life situation, may be expected to receive an objection from either Schiavo's lawyer or the judge. Instead, Terri Schiavo's menstruation, and thus, menstruation as a key element in narrativizing womanhood more broadly, is adopted as an important consideration by Michael Schiavo's lawyers as well.

Michael Schiavo's legal team, led by George Felos, also elicit evidence regarding Terri Schiavo's period. Examining Michael Schiavo, his attorney asks, "Did you and Terri ever consider having a family?" (*Schiavo* 37). Schiavo replies, "Yes. We did." After asking Michael Schiavo further questions regarding his feelings and his wife's feelings about having children, Felos asks, "Did Terri ever become pregnant?" (37) Schiavo responds, "No. She did not." Felos follows up by asking Schiavo "What was the difficulty?" to which Schiavo responds, "Terri was not receiving her period." Felos also questions Terri Schiavo's sister-in-law, asking, "You were asked a question about Terri wanting to get pregnant and seeing a doctor. Did Terri ever mention anything to you about the frequency of her periods or not getting periods?" (244). Schiavo's sister-in-law responds, "They were not real frequent."

The evidence brought forward by both sides of the case regarding Schiavo's period prior to when she became vegetative seems tangential at best and only relevant to whether or not Schiavo was previously in entirely good health, but unrelated to the decision at hand: whether or not she would want to have her life support removed. By not objecting to these lines of questioning and, in fact, by amplifying and continuing them, both sides of the case present menstruation as a key signifier in constructing Schiavo as a woman. This evidence as to Schiavo's period blood, which was heard before discussion about her desires with regard to her own life, demonstrates an accepted premise in the courtroom that menstruation, and the ways in which it is experienced, is the defining feature of women as subjects. Each side of the case builds from this scaffolding a different interpretation of what kind of woman menstrual blood establishes Schiavo to be. On one side, too much blood is presented as evidence that the female subject whose feminine processes have become publically visible is lost beyond recovery. On the other, the regularity of blood is proffered as a claim that the subject is a potential mother, who should, therefore, be preserved.

Felos's team organizes the presented evidence to support a story in which Schiavo is represented as a woman who—partly due to the overflowing nature of her heavy periods and the burden that these periods place on others—should be removed from life support. Having gathered evidence that prior to her accident Terri Schiavo "was not receiving her period," (37) George Felos questions his client about Schiavo's current health condition and about whether "Terri ha[s] a menstrual period" (260) and whether it "cause[s] any problems for her" (260). Michael Schiavo responds, "No more than any woman, but this is something that has to be attended to by the staff because she cannot care for herself" (260). Other health problems Schiavo experienced while vegetative—such as the necessity of a toe amputation, pelvic inflammatory disease, kidney stones, and several urinary tract infections so severe they required hospitalization (42)—are mentioned in passing and are not extrapolated upon to represent the extent of care needed for Schiavo and the severity of her condition. It is Terri Schiavo's menstruation that the Felos team centralizes and returns to in discussions of her condition. Felos asks Michael Schiavo the following questions:

Q. Can Terri clip her fingernails?

A. No.

Q. Comb her hair?

A. No.

Q. Can Terri dress herself?

A. No. She cannot.

Q. How are all those activities done for Terri?

A. I have her in a nursing home. The facility employees do all that for her. She has to be intubated by one person. She wears a diaper, which has to be cleaned, and you know, whether she has a BM, they have to change the diaper. Clean her. She has her period, which is at times extremely heavy and messy. They have to clean her. (*Schiavo* 41)

Schiavo's "extremely heavy and messy period" communicates to the court that menstrual blood expressed in this way and in these conditions is excessive, unnatural, and repugnant. It is significant here that Felos chooses to direct his client to focus on menstrual blood rather than the arguably more serious conditions (pelvic inflammatory disease, toe amputation, and kidney stones) mentioned above. Menstruation as the experience selected to communicate the gravity of Schiavo's medical condition—which was not objected to on grounds of irrelevance by either the judge or the opposing legal representatives—suggests that when menstrual blood is excessive and must be dealt with by others, it communicates that a woman is beyond help. This evidence, chosen above the other possible conditions to convey Schiavo's situation, also suggests a problematic assumption about women outside the courtroom. Whereas toe amputation, pelvic inflammation, and kidney stones (just a few of the complications that Schiavo, in fact, experienced) may be accepted as treatable issues that are easily handled through medical care, excessive menstrual blood, which becomes the problem of other people (specifically, of medical professionals), is understood as something also exceeding the bounds of reasonable care. Here, menstrual blood is represented as something that should be private: where it is not, where it spills from the body and must be "clean[ed]," it is evidence of a female subject who is too far gone. Having solicited evidence previously on the absence of Schiavo's period before her accident, the Felos team weaves an arc in which this lack of period is contrasted to the "extremely heavy and messy" period that followed Schiavo's vegetative state. Felos's statement, presented here again as unobjectionable evidence, suggests that when menstruation becomes a visible public act, the woman who engages in it becomes problematic to the point of being irredeemable.

Although Campbell's team may be expected to confront or dismiss Felos's rendition of menstruation, it, instead, constructs its own contrasting one around the fact that Schiavo was not menstruating prior to her accident. At the time of the trial, Schiavo had no cognitive capacities, could not move, speak, communicate, or otherwise participate in interaction with the world around her, yet the legal team representing Schiavo's parents presents her menstrual blood while vegetative as evidence that she was "just like any other woman" (395). This narrative intent becomes apparent when Campbell cross-examines Schiavo's treating physician, Dr. Gambone. Referring to the contemporary health of Schiavo as her case was being heard, nearly fifteen years after she first became vegetative, Campbell asks:

Q. Does Terri have a menstrual period?
A. Yes.

Q. Does that cause any extra problems for her?
A. No more than any woman, but this is something that has to be

attended to by the staff because she cannot care for herself. (*Schiavo* 261)

In contrast to Felos's, Campbell's rendition shows that while Schiavo might not have had periods previously, and her periods may be something that the hospital staff must take care of, the renewed presence of menstruation establishes that she is just like "any woman" (261). Campbell's interview of Mrs. Schindler follows Felos's questioning of Michael Schiavo regarding Terri Schiavo's heavy periods and reflect an effort to redirect the analysis that Felos has built around Schiavo's menstruation. Campbell asks Mrs. Schindler, "What observations do you have that would lead you to believe that she [Terri] is in pain?" (395). Mrs. Schindler responds, "Sometimes her moaning. She gets her period really, really bad and they have to give her pain pills and stuff sometimes. That way she is just like any other woman. She still has that problem" (395). In extracting this line of reasoning from her client, Campbell attempts to recontextualize the evidence that Felos has used to suggest that Schiavo's heavy periods reflect a problematic female body. Schiavo's continued menstruation is raised to demonstrate that Schiavo is an ordinary woman—whose body, exhibiting the same ordinary functions that are expected of all women—should be seen as normal, regardless of her medical condition. In her closing remarks, Campbell affirms this point as one of her central claims. Referring to Schiavo, she says the following:

> Over the last ten years, she has had hospitalizations. Most of them were in the primary time frame of right after this incident, as well as she had one female related hospitalization. Whose (sic) to know if Terri would not have had those kind of complications anyway? Jackie Rhodes testified, as well as her sister, Sue, and her mother that she regularly had female problems prior to this incident. (*Schiavo* 962)

Here, Schiavo's previous issues with her period are presented to argue that since she has always had "female problems," the fact that she still menstruates should be taken as evidence that at a basic level, her body continues to be an average "female" body; she should be treated in the same way that the court would treat any other woman, vegetative state or no. As when Felos's team presented its interpretations of Schiavo's menstrual blood, Campbell's story is not questioned. The argument that because Schiavo gets her period (for which she must take pain pills) she is like any other female (despite having been vegetative for fifteen years) could easily be objected to as information irrelevant to determining Schiavo's wishes, yet no one objects. As with the acceptance of Felos's contrasting account, this construction, and the willingness of the court to observe it, suggests an accepted discourse around menstruation beyond the Schiavo case. Although many women in society, for reasons ranging from diet to birth control use, to gender transition, do not have a menstrual period, the acceptance of Campbell's narrative suggests a commonsense understanding that to be a woman is to menstruate. Whereas Felos holds up social concerns regarding the excessive presence of menstruation, Campbell holds up concerns regarding its absence. Here, the social gesture is towards blood as evidence of so-called regular womanhood.

Campbell's final, overarching narrative draws both on this evidence and on her initial argument: Schiavo's menstrual blood is testimony that she could physically become a mother and should, therefore, be sustained on life support. During the trial, both Campbell and Felos place great emphasis on unpacking whether or not Terri Schiavo wanted to have children. In fact, where discussion of Schiavo's period occurs, it is nearly always tied to her relationship to pregnancy. This link is first initiated when Felos questions Michael Schiavo, asking whether he and his wife had wanted to have a family. When Schiavo replies that they did want children, Felos asks, "what were your feelings about that and Terri's feelings?" (37). Schiavo responds, "Terri adored children. She wanted children desperately, as I did" (37). Here, Felos affirms that Terri Schiavo's previous lack of menstruation is significant because it prevented her from having the children she desired.

Campbell builds upon this evidence through trying to affirm the connection between Schiavo's previous desire for children and her lack of menstruation while conscious. She asks Schiavo's mother, "Did you and Terri ever have conversations about she wanting to have children?" (347). Schiavo's mother responds, "I really didn't have any conversations with her about children." Campbell follows this by asking, "Did you know that she was going to a gynecologist?" to which

Mrs. Schindler responds, "I knew she was, because Terri always had problems with her period" (347). Although Mrs. Schindler cannot confirm Campbell's suggestion that Schiavo wanted children, Campbell still manages to connect Schiavo's absent period to her wish to be pregnant. She continues to assert this link through her questioning of witnesses that follow. In conversation with Schiavo's former co-worker, Jacqueline Rhodes, Campbell asks her about Schiavo's doctors' appointments, and Rhodes states the following: "I know she was having problems with her period. She said that is—she had never gotten pregnant during her and Michael's marriage and she had never been on any form of birth control. That was something she was talking to the doctor about" (805). Campbell reinforces her construction of Schiavo as a woman who "desperately" wanted but could not have children through asking "To your knowledge, did Terri become pregnant during that time frame?" Rhodes responds, "No. Not to my knowledge." Campbell asks again, "Did Terri ever indicate she was trying to have children?" Rhodes responds: "She never indicated that she wanted children. She just indicated that she had never gotten pregnant and they were looking into medically why that had not happened" (805). Campbell explicitly guides friends and family to share information regarding Schiavo's previous issues with her period and desire for children; this becomes more evident over the course of the trial.

As Campbell questions Terri Schiavo's treating physician, Dr. Gambone, she asks for the doctor's credentials and then immediately asks, "Does Terri have a menstrual period?" (261). Campbell's intention in raising Schiavo's menstruation becomes clear when she follows this by asking "Could she get pregnant?" Gambone responds, "Yes. She can" (261). In questioning Dr. Gambone, this established information is woven together with the doctor's testimony on Schiavo's heavy periods while in her vegetative state. Schiavo is established as a subject who, in fact, could potentially become a mother and, in doing so, could fulfill a previous goal that she did not achieve while conscious. Given that Terri Schiavo, at forty-one, had been vegetative for nearly fifteen years and could not give consent to sex, this line of questioning is inherently disturbing: Schiavo would have to be raped to become pregnant. Yet Felos, the judge, and the questioned witnesses do not object to it.

In Campbell's closing remarks, the assumption of Schiavo's

menstruation as evidence of her potential as a future mother is reinforced as a key piece of her argument towards keeping Terri Schiavo on life support:

> The Schindlers have testified that they believe firmly that she would choose her current medically stable life over death. That she believed in the preservation of life and that was the way she was raised. Now the Schindlers were given some visually graphic, horrible, disgusting conditions as extreme hypotheticals and asked if they would allow their daughter, Terri, to be in those circumstances beyond their imagination over death. However, Terri does not have cancer. She does not have gangrene. She does not have amputated limbs. She is not facing open heart surgery. Mr. Schindler testified that he would need to gather all the medical information needed to make such decisions. That those decisions would have to be based on the variables given at the time. Dr. Gambone testified that Terri is medically stable. She has a regular menstrual period. She could get pregnant. (*Schiavo* 961)

Although Campbell has acknowledged Schiavo's vegetative state, she presents the continuation of Schiavo's period and the fact that her body could physically become pregnant as a commonsense affirmation that Schiavo should be sustained on life support. The importance of this claim to Campbell's narrative is reinforced by its placement. After discussing hypothetical situations that would mean Schiavo was truly in a medically problematic situation, Campbell proposes that, on the contrary, Schiavo is medically well and perhaps even thriving, as evidenced by her menstruation and the physical possibility of her pregnancy.

George Felos, however, in his response to Campbell's closing remarks, argues that "there is no 'she' that knows she is having a menstrual period" (*Schiavo* 975); neither he nor the trial judge critiques the deeply flawed argument behind Campbell's insistence that Terri Schiavo "could get pregnant." Presented here, again without objection, Campbell's comments indicate a significant overarching story about menstrual blood that contains within it both of the other social stories regarding menstruation revealed in the trial. Both Felos's narrative— excessive menstrual blood witnessed and cleaned by others indicates a problematic form of womanhood—and Campbell's previous one—a normal female body bleeds—can be absorbed within the story told here: if a female body can menstruate, it can produce children.

The excessive blood, which is accepted by the court as evidence of a woman's body gone wrong, is also evidence of a body that in bleeding profusely cannot sustain motherhood. The female body that previously lacked blood begins to regularly demonstrate so-called female problems, which are managed with "pain pill ... just like any other woman" (395), and exhibits the normal processes of a body in preparation for motherhood. In Campbell's final declaration—that Schiavo's previous desire for children and her body's capability of cultivating them indicate she should be maintained on life support—there is an obvious cause for objection. Yet this assumption was not questioned when shared in a courtroom full of people: not by Felos, not by the judge, and not by the press who reported voraciously on other aspects of the trial. This tacit acceptance of the link that Campbell paints—that the potential to become pregnant should be enough in itself to demonstrate that a woman should not be granted the right to die—gestures towards a broader social acceptance of the link between menstrual blood and motherhood. Even though many women who bleed will never become mothers, by choice, by chance, or by biological potential, and even though many women who do not bleed will become mothers by other means, blood is understood to represent both the ability to have children and the desire to have children.

Following this thread, Campbell mobilizes menstruation to construct Terri Schiavo as a woman who would want to be kept on life support, not because of her feelings towards life-sustaining measures or because of her personality, values, or beliefs, but because she had wanted to have children previously and because her blood meant that her body could physically produce such children. Mobilizing evidence to suggest that even under the circumstances of an irreversible vegetative state Schiavo would still wish for a pregnancy extends a further presumption: when a woman once wanted children and when her body is still capable of delivering a pregnancy, she will wish to produce children under any circumstances. And she should be preserved for this purpose whether she is a functioning active agent or a comatose body.

By way of contrast, it is telling that in the American cases involving male patients studied by August and Miles, including those in which the men in question were in their youth, their past desires to have children, their physical capacities to be fathers, and their sperm count were never introduced as evidence for why they should be kept alive. Menstruation, as something that can be read only on a woman's body, is mobilized and accepted as a narrative tool in the Schiavo case in ways that reveal commonsense narratives about what menstrual blood says about womanhood.

In Schiavo, both legal teams cultivated graphic evidence about her menstrual cycle, how years prior she had desired children, and how "there is something in that body"(*Schiavo* 970) that would allow it to become pregnant, without anyone ever questioning the relevance of these subjects to whether Schiavo would want to remain on life support in a vegetative state. Schiavo's menstrual blood—a circumstance that is particular to her gendered body—is animated and written onto her silent body as a story by both legal teams. Schiavo is first constructed as a subject whose blood, emerging in too great a quantity, conveys that her body (and, perhaps, her life as an acceptable female subject) is irreparably lost. Accepted as it is across the courtroom and chosen to illustrate the dire nature of Schiavo's condition beyond several health crises involving hospitalization, this narrative and the acknowledgment of its validity indicate a broader social understanding of heavy menstrual blood as evidence of problematic womanhood. Schiavo is also constructed as a subject who, continuing to menstruate, can be understood to be "just like any other woman." In this story of blood, the court is encouraged to weigh the fact of Schiavo's period—absent prior to her accident but now returned and representing normal female functioning—against her medical state and to find her continued period more significant for sustaining her on life support. The acceptance of this account shows that like excessive menstrual blood, the absence of menstruation altogether speaks to the absence of life as a female subject: its return, regardless of what pain it may carry and what other issues may be read on the body, indicates femaleness restored to normal. Finally, Schiavo's menstrual blood is mobilized to construct her as a potential mother—a woman who had always wanted children and who should be sustained, despite the circumstances, for the sake of these past desires and whose blood shows they could still, at a basic level, be realized. Here, both previous narratives of blood are brought together to point to a social understanding that both excess and lack of blood highlight a body that is problematic because it is not prepared for motherhood. But in a consistently bleeding body, as Campbell argues Schiavo's has become, menstruation is understood to mean the ability to have children as well as the desire to.

As Rebecca Rausch writes, within court, "white men's bodies, straight men's gender, and upper middle class men's social position [is set as] the standard and measures all others, including women, against that norm" (35). In the eyes of the court, men with these privileges represent the ideal liberal subjects, whom federal and state constitutions, from their first iteration, recognize as participants in the political field and grant enshrined rights. Although a right to die case inevitably features a silenced body who cannot act in the political sphere, the ways in which male and female patients are constructed in these cases demonstrates the extent to which a male patient is represented and inscribed as an active agent, with his desires, previous wishes, and personality placed as paramount in making a decision. A female patient is primarily considered from the point of view of others and their relationship with her and what they consider to be in her best interests. Already removed from a debate in which her own personality, values, and beliefs are centralized by virtue of her gender, Schiavo is removed further still through the animation of her menstrual blood. In this animation, to which no one in the courtroom and no one among the public witnesses objected, blood is made to speak. Beyond the injustice of a physical signifier only being used to decipher what is right for a woman's body, the narrative threads around Schiavo's blood, raised without being challenged, operate because they represent socially accepted stories around menstruation. The way Schiavo's blood is presented in court as evidence, as well as the narratives that each legal team weaves around this blood, reflects taken-for-granted assumptions about how menstruation is experienced. Menstruation is made to speak, and it is then interpreted and expressed in limited ways through the stories told here. And although menstrual blood does not express the desire, the capability, or the means to be a mother, a socially accepted narrative of blood is gestured to in the Schiavo trial: the presence of blood is the possibility of motherhood.

Works Cited

Fiore, Robin. "Framing Terri Schiavo: Gender, Disability, and Fetal Protection." *The Case of Terri Schiavo: Ethics, Politics and Death in the 21st Century*, edited by Kenneth Goodman, Oxford University Press, 2010, pp. 191-209.

Goodman, Kenneth, editor. *The Case of Terri Schiavo: Ethics, Politics and Death in the 21st Century*. Oxford University Press, 2010.

Holloway, Karla. *Private Bodies, Public Texts: Race, Gender, and a Cultural Bioethics*. Duke University Press, 2011.

In re The Guardianship of Theresa Marie Schiavo. No. 90-2908-GD3. Circuit Court of the Sixth Judicial Circuit State of Florida in and for Pinellas County Probate Division. *Schiavo Timeline Part 1*. Schiavo Case Resources, University of Miami Ethics Programs, 2000 bioethics.miami.edu/research-and-clinical-ethics/terri-schiavo-project/schiavo-links/index.html Accessed 8 Mar. 2019.

Miles, Stephen H. and Allison August. "Courts, Gender, and the 'Right to Die.'" *Law, Medicine, and Health Care* vol. 18, no. 1-2, 1990, pp. 85-95.

Rausch, Rebecca. "Reframing Roe: Property Over Privacy." *Berkeley Journal of Gender, Law, and Justice*, vol. 27, no. 1, 2012, pp. 28-63.

Raymond, Diane. "'Fatal Practices': A Feminist Analysis of Physician-assisted Suicide and Euthanasia." *Hypatia*, vol. 14, no. 2, 1999, pp. 1-25.

Chapter Three

Period Porn: Menstrual Blood at the Margins

Laura Helen Marks

"So we can just shove any food we want into our asses but period blood isn't allowed in porn right"—tweet from Janice Griffith, @thejanicexxx, 26 Nov. 2016

Some years ago, I came across a thread on an adult film forum I frequent in which a user, bi_girl, asked for menstrual porn recommendations. She was promptly accused of being a troll. In response, bi_girl wrote the following:

I'm not joking :(. Is it that unfathomable that someone might be turned on by a woman who is on her period? Has no chick ever had an orgasm while they were on their period, masturbating, having sex, otherwise? I see it as no more bizarre than a double anal creampie snowballing, painful anal, "dirty ass to mouth," or even incest fetish, all of which I've seen on this forum. So please, don't be so judgmental. I asked an honest question.

Months later, while writing a chapter on hardcore adaptations of *Dracula*, I was somewhat surprised that no pornographers had taken advantage of the sexual potential of menstrual blood in a vampire film. This prompted me to consider what porn—that genre where everything and anything goes and where excess and the transgression of social norms are the ostensible generic function—finds to be obscene within its own codes of representation. In a genre that claims to speak the unspoken and revel in social taboo, menstrual blood holds a unique place as the one truly obscene representation; that is, off scene. In this sense, although feces, urine, and interspecies sex may be regarded as profoundly taboo and certainly not part of mainstream pornography, even these niche subgenres are indeed *subgenres* with names recognizable even to those who have never come across this type of content: scat, watersports, and bestiality or "zoo" porn, respectively. Pornography is a genre of media that supposedly locates "each and every one of society's taboos, prohibitions, and proprieties and systematically transgress[es] them, one by one" (Kipnis 164). Menstrual blood—its absence, its appearance, and its reappearance— is a handy indicator of those particular areas where pornography and its consumers (and by extension society as a whole) fear to tread.

Menstruation stigma and taboo have been well documented in feminist scholarship. Via advertisements, socialization, and everyday discourse, menstruation is conveyed as "a 'hygienic crisis' that must be concealed and managed" (Goldenberg and Roberts 75). The menstruating woman is stigmatized, and is prompted to engage in rituals of cleansing and concealment (Johnston-Robledo and Chrisler 10). More recently, however, Breanne Fahs has explored the anarchist, DIY response to such cultural attitudes. The existence of menstruation is more visible in porn and its paratexts than people assume. Indeed, menstrual blood might be considered, to use Linda Williams's term, "on/scene." On/scenity, Williams describes, is:

> The more conflicted term with which we can mark the tension between the speakable and the unspeakable which animates so many of our contemporary discourses of sexuality... On/scenity is thus an ongoing negotiation that produces increased awareness of those once-obscene matters that now peek at us from under every bush. ("Porn Studies" 4-5)

In the case of menstrual blood and pornography, as I show here, the paratexts of porn constitute these "bushes"—menstrual blood seeps into the marginal texts and incidental moments at the periphery of what we are told is the main event. In actuality, paratexts of porn are integral components of pornographic pleasure. I contend that in their peripheral status, paratexts constitute exciting components of the main text and accrue special sexual properties due to a transgressive sense of being both on and off scene.

Outside of menstrual-themed porn, tampons are referenced in plot points. Periods occur with no forewarning or labelling on the video; periods are discussed in behind-the-scenes segments, and porn stars talk about their periods on blogs, in interviews, and in tweets. Adding to the complexity of this situation, menstrual blood has been taken up by feminist pornographers as a way to challenge sexist double standards as well as by more male-oriented pornographers capitalizing on the so-called extreme nature of menstrual porn.

In the subsequent chapter, I argue that period blood occupies a unique place among bodily fluids in film, video, photographic, and online pornographies. The relative absence of menstrual blood in porn signals two interrelated perspectives: one of misogynistic disgust towards menstruation and one of fear and discomfort at the sight of blood in porn. I believe that although menstrual blood is, indeed, considered a taboo within porn, the surrounding paratexts—behind-the-scenes footage, blogs, and interviews—are rich repositories for menstrual representation. Moreover, in contrast to the fetishized pornographic representations of menstruation typically found in menstrual-themed porn, paratextual representations of menstruating bodies have a normalizing effect. Simultaneously absent and present, menstrual blood has a particular transgressive currency in hardcore, symbolic of the extreme, the obscene, and the authentic. Drawing on theories of the paratext and the abject, I explore the special regulating forces that shape what can and cannot be shown in particular pornographic media, in particular pornographic contexts. Through this analysis, I locate the pornographic paratext as a productive site of subversion and as indicative of the displaced erotics and authenticating power of menstruation.

Transgression, Authenticity, and Desire

Transgression and authenticity are integral parts of pornographic pleasure and arousal. When I refer to "pleasure and arousal," I mean the particular "resonance," as Susanna Paasonen describes it, which "has no predictable direction or trajectory" and which may include registers of disgust, intrigue, and shock alongside the more traditional understandings of genital arousal (Paasonen 17). Writing in 1996, Laura Kipnis argues that pornography is "a form of political theater [and] within the incipient, transgressive space opened by its festival of social infractions is a medium for confronting its audiences with exactly those contents that are exiled from sanctioned speech, from mainstream culture and political discourse. And that encompasses more than sex" (164). In a digital pornographic age, Kipnis's argument has only accrued greater relevance.

In the Internet age, transgression and authenticity function in complex ways that interact with technology to generate particular erotic appeal. Paasonen observes the following:

> Pornographic images and videos involve a complex interplay between authenticity and artifice, the indexical and the hyperbolic, immediacy and distance. At the heart of this interplay lies the physical presence and visual accessibility of its performers, facilitated by networked communications and supported by the notions of realness and authenticity associated with technologies of inscription, imaging, recording, and transmission (via photography, video, and the Internet). Such "carnal residue" is crucial to the affective registers, force, and appeal of online porn. (17)

The mining of celebrities' private lives for videotaped or photographed sexual activity—whether through hacking as in the case of Jennifer Lawrence and others targeted by the so-called fappening or through contracted performance as in the case of pro-wrestler Chyna and reality television star Farrah Abraham who made reality porn tapes for Vivid Video— suggests that consumers find the exposure of (female) private sex lives endlessly fascinating and titillating (Lawson 607). In the case of porn stars, however, consumers have ready access to their sexual practices. The impulse to see something authentically sexual remains, however, evidenced in series such as *Chemistry* (Dir. Tristan Taormino, 2006-2008) and *Raw* (Dir. Manuel Ferrara, 2009-present) that attempt to document candid, authentic sexual activity between professional pornographic performers.

Menstrual blood, however, stands in contrast to these represent-ations of authentic sexuality. Menstrual blood is taboo and undocumented even in advertising and everyday conversation. Menstrual blood is, perhaps, the most secret of practices related to female genitalia, sexuality, and orifices, and thus carries a special signification when it comes to authenticity and female bodies. In this way, paratextual pornographic menstrual blood is especially transgressive and constitutes a form of what Fahs calls a "highly gendered form of graffiti" (34). Pornographers who deploy menstrual blood in their paratextual representations perform a particularly powerful "bleeding through ... giving language to their menstrual blood that has crossed a barrier, pushed through a boundary, ruptured the existing social order" (Fahs 38)—powerful in that they harness the erotic to the menstrual, a combination particularly offensive to social norms. Paratextual pornographic menstruation promises visual access to that most discreet of female corporeal processes, and thus it holds a special form of transgressive eroticism through this very access.

Abject Fluids and Pornography

The most logical explanation for the absence of menstrual blood in porn is that menstrual blood has a special abject status among other abject fluids. This special status is very much tied to its relation to the female body; thus, the absence of menstrual blood in porn is understandably interpreted as a misogynistic absence symbolic of societal disgust towards female bodies and their contents. As Julia Kristeva argues, abject bodily fluids such as vomit, semen, saliva, and blood inspire disgust and anxiety because they transgress the borders of inside/outside, threatening the (illusory) sense of a unified, contained, and controlled self (53).

Bodily fluids and the scant control we have over them is a source of fear and anxiety. Disgust mobilizes our rejection of these fluids, pushing them away from our body to maintain the illusion that we are whole. At the same time, abject bodily fluids engender desire for the gooey, warm interior of the womb. In a more concrete sense, as evidenced by our childhood activities and, when permitted, those of adulthood, getting messy is necessary in establishing borders and shoring up identity. It is also both fascinating and fun. Pornography is a primary site where these contradictory feelings happily merge. It incorporates a multitude of abject fluids. Semen, saliva, mucous, female ejaculate, enema water, urine, and vomit are just a few that are either so ubiquitous they are seemingly compulsory (semen) or less common but nevertheless quite visible in even mainstream porn (vomit).[1] Considering the plethora of abject fluids, the relative absence of menstrual blood is worth interrogating. Tanya Krzywinska argues that "most hardcore couches bodily fluids and the organs that produce them within the framework of sexual transgression so that the substances can be secret(e)ly experienced in a pleasurable way" (38). Not all abject fluids are equal, though. According to Kristeva, the reproductive and nourishing fluids—milk and semen—are the least disgusting while bodily waste is the most disgusting.

The narrative surrounding particular fluids appears to influence which are represented with the most gusto in pornography. Semen enjoys a near mythical status thanks to centuries of folklore (including pornography) that valorize this magical substance and hold it in awe. As discussed by Linda Williams in *Hard Core*, among other scholars, the "money shot"—ejaculation onto the man's or woman's body—is perhaps the most compulsively prerequisite feature of the hardcore pornographic genre, particularly the heterosexual variety. The money shot, Williams contends, is hardcore's striving for "maximum visibility" (94) and "visual evidence of the mechanical 'truth' of bodily pleasure" (101). However, as Williams notes, this "ultimate ... confession of sexual pleasure" only speaks to male sexual pleasure (119).

Perhaps menstrual blood is too abject or too connotative of violence and death, while semen connotes life, creation, and reassures the masculine self (Kristeva 53). Blood rests at what Julia Kristeva calls a "fascinating semantic crossroads": "the propitious place for abjection, where *death* and *femininity, murder* and *procreation, cessation of life* and *vitality* all come together" (62). But there is also undoubtedly a gendered element at work here:

> Neither tears nor sperm ... although they belong to borders of the body, have any polluting value ... Menstrual blood ... stands for the danger issuing from within the identity (social and sexual); it threatens the relationship between the sexes within a social aggregate and, through internalization, the identity of each sex in the face of sexual difference. (Kristeva 71)

Whereas excess semen mitigates against masculine crisis in that it suggests the fluids emanating from the male body are appealing and desirable, menstrual blood is received as a threat to the masculine subject—as gross, as alien, and as irretrievably female.

The lack of menstrual porn, and the disgust directed towards menstrual blood in general, would appear to support Kristeva's argument. Indeed, it does to a great extent. The argument I make here about paratextual recovery of menstrual fluid does not exclude the contention that society regards menstruation as shameful and dirty or that this attitude is rooted in misogyny. But, instead, I hope to unfold the ways in which these misogynistic attitudes of disgust and subsequent absence of menstrual porn lead to gestures of defiance and revelation at the margins of pornography. Although menstrual-themed porn certainly exists, I am interested in how the pornographic paratext draws on the generic drive for authenticity resulting in dynamic paratextual representations of periods that invest the text with additional meaning, normalize menstruating bodies, and engage with the erotics of menstruation.

Related to horror and disgust towards the female body and its fluids, a major reason pornographers give for not including menstrual blood in their films is draconian payment processors who typically refuse to process payments for content deemed "high risk" (Alptraum)—that is, content that edges into the realm of that subjective category, "the obscene," and is, thus, potentially troubling from a legal standpoint. Fears of obscenity charges have long shaped pornographic content. High-risk material may include urination and other forms of bodily waste, fisting (constituting violence), or representations of non-consent. Menstrual blood falls under the high-risk category because blood as a whole is deemed high risk. Such regulation appears to be rooted in a sexist (mis)understanding of menstrual blood as a form of bodily waste, akin to feces, as well as a symbol of violence. For example, in 2005 *BloodyTrixie*'s payment processor, Verotel, suspended their account, explaining the reason as such:

Today we unfortunately had to suspend your account. In October last year we had a content policy change. No sites with blood on them were allowed form [sic] that time on. In [the] first instance, blood in combination with violence was the main issue. However now also the sites you have can't process with us anymore. As the sites completely focus on the blood, I don't see an option to keep us processing for them. ("Join")

As Lux Alptraum observes, such a view "upholds the notion that women's bodies are shameful, and that vaginas and the things that come out of them are dirty." However, payment processors are also nervous about pornographic content depicting violence. Alptraum reports that Colin Rowntree of BDSM site *Wasteland.com* was made to stop using red wax because "payment processors seem to think melted red wax is a dead ringer for blood" (qtd. in Alptraum). Menstrual blood thus occupies a uniquely problematic place in pornography. On the one hand, it is (wrongly) viewed as bodily waste, and on the other hand, it resembles the product of physical trauma. This latter reason also plays a role in why viewers may find unlabelled, unannounced menstrual blood unsettling and a turn off. Although it is undoubtedly true that many porn viewers simply find menstrual blood gross, other viewers simply find the sight of blood emanating from an orifice in porn to be alarming, prompting concern for the female performer, particularly if the film does not clarify the nature of the blood through categorization or title. In a review of *Bordello Blues*, YogaGrrl notes, "It also bothers me to see a drop of blood clinging to Renee's perineum while they do anal doggie. Hopefully, it's only menstrual blood (since she doesn't seem to be in pain), but it almost looks like it's dribbling out of her anus." Responses such as this one suggest that distaste for menstrual blood in porn may not always be the result of misogynistic disgust.

Paratextual Pornographies

The paratext, as Gérard Genette outlined in his influential *Seuils*, is "the reinforcement and accompaniment of a certain number of productions [that] surround [the text] and prolong it, precisely in order to *present* it" (261). The function of the paratext, according to Genette, is to promote, advance, and in general offer up the text to a consuming public. In the years since Genette's coining of "paratext," media have proliferated on a profound level. Pornography in particular has generated a wide array of different paratexts that are intimately tied to the primary text in ways specific to the genre. For example, with the rise of porn that deemphasizes traditional narrative and instead rhetorically claims to represent reality and authenticity, scenes are commonly bookended by interviews with the performers. DVDs provide behind-the-scenes featurettes, and newly restored classics offer director commentaries and interviews. In the Internet era, porn stars manage their personas online in a dynamic straddling of on-screen and off-screen personality. Fans candidly discuss the taboo subject of hardcore and engage with industry professionals to request stars, offer feedback, and conduct interviews. Moreover, texts are fragmented, retitled, categorized, and uploaded to tube sites, while the official sites provide comment threads and discussion forums for viewers to leave their thoughts.[2]

Discussing the paratexts of *Pornhub*, a popular tube site, Rebecca Inez Saunders observes that the interviews that bookend scenes "rarely propose contradictory interpretations of the film" (241). Indeed, this claim could be levelled at all pornographic paratexts—after all, they are in part marketing materials. However, although these paratexts must be regarded as constructed materials designed to accompany a primary text, it is also important to take pornography's insistence on authenticity into account, particularly as far as performer voices go. As Saunders notes, the "growing tendency in film and television to provide extra-diegetic bonus materials ... together with concerns regarding the veracity of female pleasure, has seen female porn performers increasingly encouraged to talk about their experiences within the film itself" (24). This representational authenticity means that although much of this talk is certainly designed to assure the viewer of the performer's consent (as in interviews for *Kink.com* in which performers describe what they enjoyed about the scene) or to craft a fantasy of sexual spontaneity (as in the various behind-the-scenes segments that appear to show performers having sex off camera for fun), paratextual materials do often contradict or complicate the film or scene in question. Due in part to the drive for authenticity, pornographic paratexts often contain the materials that the finished porn text regards as taboo, resulting in a complicated set of extra-diegetic discourse, which is designed not only to market and promote but also to surprise and defy.

Hardcore Menstrual Narratives

Despite the supposed taboo against menstrual blood in porn, there are a handful of menstrual-themed sites such as *MenstruationSluts*, *BloodyTrixie*, and *EroticRed*, as well as some out of print menstrual DVD titles. These menstrual-themed primary texts fetishizing and focusing on menstruation as an erotic and arousing (as well as disgusting) event are not the focus of this essay. Rather, I am interested in the incidents of menstrual blood that slip through the cracks, go unnoticed, or are otherwise marginal to but couched within the mainstream porn industry.[3] Menstrual blood and menstrual materials do occasionally crop up unexpectedly in porn that is not menstrual themed. This presence of menstrual blood at the margins of porn not only suggests what is deemed too gross for porn but also demonstrates the illicit titillation of menstruation.

Menstrual blood in pornography was as elusive in the 1970s as it is now—more so, in fact, thanks to the underdeveloped nature of the industry and pre-Internet production and distribution methods. Thus, compared to today's digitally proliferating perversions, there was a lack of established micro-fetishes and categories. Menstruation cropped up in some early loops (one-reel pornographic films), serving as central themes in titles such as *Tampon Rapist* and *Tampon Freak*. Even with these titles, however, the menstruation itself is not the focal point; the materials signifying menstrual blood are. Indeed, early features quite helpfully highlight the way menstruation is framed as an off screen event, something accidental or in need of navigation, even when it is ostensibly part of the narrative. From the early days of the modern porn film industry, menstruation has been deployed as a symbol of authenticity. In 1971's *Blue Money*, for example, a film that details the fictional adventures of a married pornographer, one of the female performers working on the protagonist's set gets her period and filming must halt. Menstruation is utilized as a way to show the ins and outs of porn filmmaking, right down to the inconveniences and messy details.

In Alex DeRenzy's 1970 white coater (a pornographic film masquer-ading as a documentary so as to get away with showing unsimulated sex) *Sexual Encounter Group*, a quite startling instance of spontaneous menstrual blood occurs during the concluding orgy. The film is shot in a naturalistic style, seeming to occur in real time with very few edits.

DeRenzy's camera floats through the crowd, hovering over or zooming in on particular participants. At one point, DeRenzy zooms in on a dismounting woman to reveal a penis lightly coated in blood. As the camera backs up a little, we see the male owner of said penis, looking a little shocked, gingerly (and rather ineffectively) wiping the blood off with his hand. He and his sexual partner take a short break before he resumes intercourse with a different woman. As opposed to halting the shoot as in *Blue Money*, DeRenzy emphasizes the documentary authenticity by not shying away from this spontaneous moment. Indeed, the appearance of menstrual blood merely bolsters the authenticity and truth telling of the documentary. It is no coincidence that these early examples of menstrual blood in porn are both texts that claim forms of truth telling—one telling the behind-the-scenes story of porn filmmaking and the other telling the truths of group sex and bodies. In these two contrasting examples, menstrual blood serves as an authenticating symbol.

Another way pornographers have integrated menstrual blood into the film's narrative is through the promotional materials surrounding the text. For the marketing surrounding *Live in My Secrets*, director and star Kimberly Kane articulates spectral imaginings of menstrual blood—menstrual blood that does not appear in the actual film. In the final scene of the film, "Blood," Kane and Sasha Grey engage in a variety of sex acts covered in what appears to be blood, but which is explicitly shown to be strawberry syrup. Still, Kane points out in the commentary and in other promotional materials that Grey was menstruating during filming and did not use a sponge: "She was actually on her period in this scene, so I was like don't put in a sponge or anything, just bleed, you know, just bleed. I'll like it. So during shooting she'd be like oh, see that string? That's really blood! And I'm like oh, hot, I'll lick it off." Yet, Kane is sure to conspicuously cut to and zoom in on the empty bottle of strawberry syrup on the ground as if to make patently clear that this is a simulation. The strawberry syrup stands in for menstrual blood, conjuring the potential erotics of menstruation without actually including it. In turn, the promise made in the paratextual materials that somewhere amid all the syrup—impossible to see—is actual menstrual blood mobilizes these erotics through ambiguity. The viewer can indulge in a simulation while teetering on the "is it or isn't it?" fantasy generated by the paratext.

The force and appeal of marginal, paratextual, and spontaneous pornographic representation are rooted in spectatorial desire for a fleeting moment of unorthodox imagery or an anticipated glimpse of something outside of the norm of visual representation. The search, the moment of discovery, and the recording of that moment for personal and shared use are important aspects of erotic engagement with pornography. Porn consumers are active participants. The search, the click, the screen grab, and the logging of information can all be considered part of twenty-first century pornographic consumption (Paasonen 177-179). There is erotic appeal in witnessing a fleeting moment of reality, an accidental discovery, and the subsequent recording and documentation of that moment. This enjoyment is heightened when the image or act in question is difficult to find or taboo. Fans enjoy time stamping fleeting moments of interest in a detailed, obsessive, and committed way that moves beyond simple sharing of information and into bibliophilic erotic engagement akin to the obsessive taxonomy of the nineteenth century.[4] The more committed users even take screenshots that detail the seconds-long incidents in minute detail and offer commentary.[5] The discovery of menstrual blood in paratexts or incidental pornographic moments can carry the same erotic excitement of access, authenticity, and transgressive titillation.

Fantasies of discovery are present in some reviews of Kane's film, which highlight the ambiguous play between blood and syrup and which Kane includes in the marketing rhetoric. One reviewer of the film notes their wish that the scene went further and appears to erotically indulge in the possibilities that real blood may be involved:

I must be really dirty because I was dying to see Sasha's period blood, and to see Kimberly lap it up. Of course, that never happened, and things stayed relatively tame. There is something to be said, however, about how both women lose themselves in each other, with no toys except for the blood. Kimberly calls this scene a display of "honest sexuality." (qtd. in Epiphora)

This reviewer evidently enjoys the fantasy of real blood and is erotically invested in the anticipation of perhaps glimpsing real blood. She also finds erotic appeal in the "dirtiness" of her desires—an erotic appeal that exists regardless of whether actual menstrual blood was involved or can be seen. The rhetoric of paratexts, such as this review, and Kane's promotional rhetoric demonstrate the extent to which pornographers may use fantastical, fake representations of menstrual blood as a way to invite the erotic pleasures that menstrual blood—or the idea of it—can invoke.

In an interesting paratextual example, Howard Ziehm reveals in a 2016 DVD commentary heretofore unnoticed menstrual blood in a scene from his 1979 film, *Star Virgin*. The scene depicts a 1950s Garden of Eden in which Adam and Eve use a variety of fruits as part of their intercourse, grotesquely mashing the fruit against their bodies (and inside hers) and consuming it. During a moment where Adam penetrates Eve's vagina with a peeled banana, Ziehm observes in the commentary that "when he pulls it out he notices she's on her period ... and being the good actor that he is ... [Bud Wise] does a momentary take and then eats the banana." Now that Ziehm points it out, it is evident there is a very slight red tinge on the tip of the banana and Wise does pause for a second to look at it before enthusiastically stuffing it in his mouth. He then moves on to a bout of committed cunnilingus. Without the director commentary, the menstrual blood would likely never be noticed. This belated paratext reinserts menstrual blood in a scene that previously was thought to have none, altering not only the moment in which the blood is seen but also the sexual activities surrounding it. Moreover, this paratext reveals a candid moment for the actors constituting a silent discourse on menstrual blood that affirms its unexceptional nature and perhaps even demonstrates its erotic charge.

Bleeding Behind the Scenes

In delineating the limits of pornographic transgression in behind-the-scenes content, Sanna Härmä and Joakim Stolpe erroneously claim that, "even in behind-the-scenes materials that are fascinated with bodily fluids, there is no menstrual blood" (118). As my argument here demonstrates, although it is true that in comparison to other bodily fluids, menstruation is rarely depicted in behind-the-scenes material, it is not entirely absent. In fact, as I argue here, behind-the-scenes materials and other paratexts are quite bountiful spaces for candid representations of menstruation and menstruating bodies.

Typically, menstrual blood is edited out, soaked up with sea sponges, or quickly removed with a trusty baby wipe. These moments are invisible in the finished product but are very visible in porn's surrounding paratexts. In this way, although the separation of menstrual blood from the product proper signals the taboo, unappealing status of menstrual blood and the menstruating body, these paratexts simultaneously offer imagery of menstruation as a normal part of the porn workplace and production process. In the Showtime reality television show *Deeper Throat*, which chronicled the making of Vivid's *Throat: A Cautionary Tale* (2008), Evan Stone performs a scene with Sasha Grey while she is menstruating, and they cut to wipe a trickle of blood from her upper thigh. Any viewer of this series can then see the edited sex scene in question through a new lens—viewing the scene (rightfully) as one involving a menstruating woman even though the menstrual blood is never seen or referred to in the finished product. The interplay between the seen and the unseen, the on scene and the off scene, is crucial to pornographic eroticism. Knowledge of the paratextual reality—the off scene representation—augments the on scene representation with a sense of knowing that heightens eroticism.

Another example of paratextual menstruation in porn is a photo set titled "On My Period," published in 2004 to the now defunct *EnterBelladonna* website, run by porn star and director Belladonna and her husband Aiden Riley.[6] Typically, hardcore websites run photo sets to accompany a scene. However, Belladonna offered a long running series of behind-the-scenes photo sets under a section called "Captured." This section framed the shots as spontaneous and involved more intimate activities, such as urination. The photo set serves as a curious form of paratext. In a world of pornography where video is king and still photos are increasingly obsolete, this menstrual photo set can usefully be regarded as the paratext to a film that could never be. Moreover, the photographs are intimate and bereft of the glossy and photoshopped sheen one might expect from a porn site. In some pictures, Belladonna is shown smiling at the camera with blood on her fingertips; in some, she is tasting the blood, while in others, all we can see is her genital area as she squats over a toilet, vulva red and spread, blood suspended in a dark string (see figure 1).

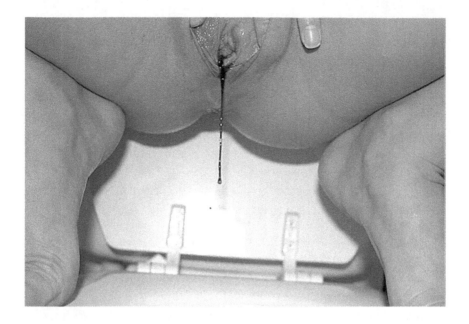

In three standalone menstrual images posted to the same section of the site, Belladonna captions the pictures in candid fashion: "Bleeding is annoying," "His load mixed with mine," and in reference to a diva cup she is messily extracting from her vagina, "This shit doesn't work. Don't waste your money." In this way, the photo set and standalone images appear to offer a glimpse into the real sexual life and everyday bodily functions of Belladonna, with menstruation the ultimate in authenticating evidence.

The media themselves carry erotic weight. Belladonna's candid photographs, the handheld, seemingly spontaneous behind-the-scenes documentation, and the first-person interviews and testimonials—all contribute to a technologically produced authenticity. The images and descriptions are mediated at a distance, yet the bodies feel amateur, spontaneous, and present. As Paasonen explains, the amateurish or spontaneous images "resonate in a mundane and intimate mode that invites a curious and titillating gaze but does not allow a comfortable sense of distance. Such closeness can be sensed as disturbing, but it is also where much of the attraction of the amateur imaging lies" (105). Such erotic closeness is also generated in porn discourses, such as interviews, porn star blogs, and Twitter feeds.

Social media discourses are rich repositories of menstrual blood in porn, or they serve as commentary on its absence. Off set, porn stars are quite forthcoming about the various ways they navigate their cycle. The primary method of working while on one's period is with the sea sponge. In her *Reddit* "Ask Me Anything" (AMA), porn star Siri states, "I was most surprised to find out that *all female performers* are expected to work as usual while on their periods. And the industry's incredibly elegant solution to prevent a girl from creating a bloody mess on film? Shove makeup sponges up your vagina to block the flow of blood" ("I Am Siri," emphasis in original). Likewise, Stoya explains the following in an interview for the podcast *Guys We Fucked*:

> So you put a boiled sponge in there, but first you get the bottle of douche and you dump that out, because ... you need to rinse the blood out first. So you dump out what's in the douche bottle, you rinse it out in the sink ... then you take freezing fucking cold ice water, dump it into the douche bottle, make sure everyone on set is ready to go. And then you're in the bathroom, ice water, shove the sponge in, run to set, and then you go for as long as you can, and the other performer or performers and the camera operator and all that will be keeping an eye out because eventually more blood than the sponge can soak up happens, and then so you have to cut [the scene] because you can't show that. ("The Stoya Episode")

You "can't show that" in the finished, edited product, but you can show that or describe that in paratextual media surrounding the film. Not only do these behind-the-scenes texts—interviews, blog posts, and featurettes—reveal the normalcy and ever presentness of menstruation in porn, they also demonstrate the comfort with which all parties involved—director, photographer, co-star, etc.—handle menstrual blood. In the *Throat* outtakes depicted in the Showtime series, for example, Evan Stone is unfazed by the constant cutting to wipe blood from his penis. He can be seen patiently waiting on his back, penis erect and ready.

Performer Christian X demonstrates this comfort bordering on celebration on his blog *Christian Sings the Blues*, where he details his daily work in porn as a performer and director. In a post from 2008, he describes a scene with Esperanza Diaz, remarking, "Oh yes, as an added bonus I get to gross out at least half of my readers by getting to pull her sponges out after the scene. Good times!" Included in this post is a series of photos detailing the sponge extraction, concluding with a close up of the faintly brownish-red sponge ("She's Definitely a Big Deal") (see figure 2).

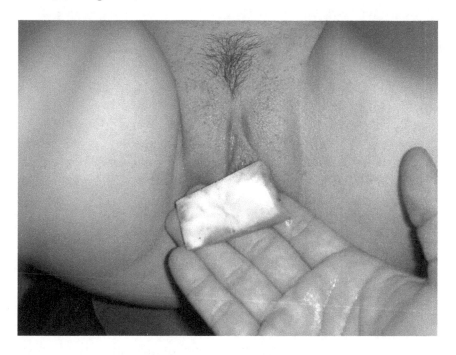

Christian's remark indicates an amused understanding that menstrual blood is simply part of his job and something that does not bother him at all, whereas his civilian readers unfamiliar with the life of a porn star will likely be grossed out—an affective experience that intersects with pleasure and arousal.

The advanced attitudes of porn stars—attitudes cultivated by the conditions of employment—are also on display in a *Nerve* article, "This Is Why We Should Embrace Period Sex," in which porn star Wolf Hudson is turned to as an expert on the subject. Hudson advises, "As a precaution, if she's experiencing a heavy flow and it's stressing her out during sex, I always keep makeup sponges handy as they're super absorbent for such an event" (qtd. in Seale). In these diverse paratexts, porn is configured as a space where menstruation is no big deal as well as something that indicates revelation and authenticity. Even though the finished, edited products of porn are typically scrubbed clean of blood (as is vomit and feces, for the most part), they are also augmented by porn star revelations of the standard workplace status of menstruation.

Menstruation in porn may be relegated in most cases to behind the scenes, interviews, commentaries, and other locations outside of the primary text, but its inclusion in paratextual material reveals the erotics of menstruation through a sublimated representation. Menstruation must be sequestered, but it is still there. It appears that erotic enjoyment of menstruation and the various illicit thrills it generates must occur a step away from a direct address due to legal and logistic restrictions, which in turn create an abject space in which a transgressive sense of erotic authenticity can be enjoyed. These paratextual spaces offer up material that is pornographic but also not the main event. These spaces are staged in such a way as to make them authentic and real and, thus, more exciting in their transgressive peek behind the curtain. Menstruation is a valuable currency in this particular paratextual space. As the most taboo of the bodily fluids, it is a particularly profound marker of authenticity and "what really goes on." The potential disgust menstrual porn may provoke is mediated by the framework of the paratext—this is not porn. It is both/and porn, not either/or. Instead, the viewer gets a privileged look at not only what happens between shoots and during breaks but also what these starlets really get up to on their down time. In this way, porn paratexts highlight the abject status of menstrual blood in specific pornographic contexts while defusing this abject status in other contexts. These paratexts collectively augment the sterilized and edited porn text; they normalize menstruation at the same time as they re-emphasize the stringent removal of menstruation from porn. The existence of menstruation in these forms complicates the straightforward reading of menstrual absence as a misogynistic, disgusted reaction to the abject female body. Instead, while rarely depicted head on or in the same quantities as semen, saliva, and bile, menstruation is, nevertheless, present in peripheral form. In these peripheral moments, menstruation announces its typically silenced or ignored erotic qualities.

Endnotes

1. *Hookup Hotshot* shows deep throating to the point of vomit. The site also features urination. Significantly, site owner, director, and performer Bryan Gozzling has indicated that he has had to cut some of the vomit and urine in scenes that are co-hosted by popular gonzo ("reality" style porn that acknowledges the camera) site *Evil Angel*. Nevertheless, even the Evil Angel edits depict large quantities of stringy, white fluid. Whether this is vomit or not is subjective. See the thread, "Bryan Gozzling Evil Angel Hookup Hotshot" on *AdultDVDTalk*. For carefully documented instances of vomiting in porn, see the thread, "Girls Puking Saliva during Blowjob," also on *AdultDVDTalk*. For a scholarly analysis of gagging and puking in porn including several mainstream porn titles that feature these acts, see Hester, "Exchanging Bodily Fluids."

2. Studios that regularly include pre- and post-scene interviews with the performers include *Kink and HardX*. Of particular note, Mason, currently director for *HardX*, features extensive interviews with performers. See for example, *Tori Black Is Pretty Filthy* (2009), *Dani Daniels: Dare* (2012), *Keisha* (2014), *Mia* (2016), and *Abella* (2016). Restored classic porn is currently enjoying a moment. The most prolific company restoring classic porn is Vinegar Syndrome. They put out HD restorations of 1970s and 1980s adult film with bonus materials, such as director and performer interviews and commentaries. *AdultDVDTalk* is the primary fan forum for discussion of porn. The site includes reviews, interviews, and porn industry engagement in discussion threads. The site also offers a chat room where performers, directors, and industry affiliates have appeared to interact with fans. Other fan forums include *Vintage Erotica Forum* and *FreeOnes*. To my knowledge, all official sites host comment threads. For a particularly engaged example, see *Pornfidelity*, which proudly declares on its homepage, "Tell us what you think! Submit your comments in the 'Your Opinion' box that's located on every episode page above the Flash player." It also hosts daily polls and offers email addresses of the site owners and performers Ryan and Kelly Madison; they state they will read and respond to each and every email.

3. By "mainstream," I mean pornographic content that is easily available on leading streaming and DVD sites or more generally any content that is not deemed a specialty item (such as urination), legally risky (such as bondage that draws blood), or outright illegal (such as bestiality, even though bestiality's legal status is a grey area in some states). What constitutes "mainstream," "indie," and "specialty" or "fetish" porn is difficult to pin down to say the least, and I will not attempt to make rigid definitions here. Menstrual porn is considered both as a specialty and as legally risky; thus, I do not classify it as mainstream. Indeed, as I discuss above, *BloodyTrixie* has shut down due to the inability to secure a payment processor, while *MenstruationSluts* and *EroticRed* appear to be dormant. All of the DVD titles are out of print, and the majority are impossible to find. The one title I could secure, Rag Time Red 6, cost me the exorbitant price of $60, and for a used copy. The titles and websites discussed in this chapter are not menstrual themed and are thus not considered a specialty. They are all in print and widely available, except for *EnterBelladonna*, which shut down midway through writing this chapter. For this reason, and for want of a better term, I describe the titles as mainstream.

4. See Steven Marcus, *The Other Victorians: A Study of Sexuality and Pornography in Mid-Nineteenth-Century England*. See also the biography of famed bibliophile Henry Spencer Ashbee, *Erotomaniac: The Life of Henry Spencer Ashbee* by Ian Gibson.

5. See, for example, the following threads on AdultDVDTalk: "Unplanned Anal Scenes" (https://forum.adultdvdtalk.com/just-a-little-bit-of-anal), "Dirty A2M & Messy Anal -Bloopers & Unexpected Leak," (https://forum.adultdvdtalk.com/dirty-a2m-messy-anal-bloopers-unexpected-leak), and "Girls Puking Saliva During Blowjob" (https://forum.adultdvdtalk.com/girls-puking-saliva-during-blowjob).

6. I am indebted to Karl of *yesterdayserotic.tumblr.com* (an impressive archive of online watersports content). *EnterBelladonna* shut down midway through writing this chapter. Karl provided me with the entire set of photos as well as vital contextual information.

Works Cited

Alptraum, Lux. "The Secret Censorship of Online Porn." *Motherboard*, 25 Nov. 2015, motherboard.vice.com/en_us/article/kb7ak9/the-secret-censorship-of-online-porn. Accessed 26 Feb. 2019.

bi_girl. "Period Porn." *AdultDVDTalk*, 22 Jan. 2010, forum.adult dvdtalk.com/period-porn-145410. Accessed 26 Feb. 2019.

Blue Money. Directed by Alain Patrick, Vinegar Syndrome, 2017.

Epiphora. *"Review: Live in My Secrets." XCritic*, 8 Feb. 2009, https://heyepiphora.com/2009/02/review-live-in-my-secrets/ Accessed 4 Mar. 2019.

Fahs, Breanne. *Out for Blood: Essays on Menstruation and Resistance.* SUNY, 2016.

Genette, Gérard. "Introduction to the Paratext." *New Literary History*, vol. 22, no. 2 Spring 1991, pp. 261-272.

Goldenberg, Jamie L. and Tomi-Ann Roberts. "The Beast within the Beauty: An Existential Perspective on the Objectification and Condemnation of Women." *Handbook of Experimental Psychology*, edited Jeff Greenberg et al., Guildford, 2004, pp. 71-85.

Härmä, Sanna, and Joakim Stolpe. "Behind the Scenes of Straight Pleasure." *Porn.com: Making Sense of Online Pornography*, edited by Feona Attwood, Peter Lang, 2010, pp. 107-122.

Hester, Helen. "Exchanging Bodily Fluids: Transubstantiations in Contemporary Pornography." *A Journal of Queer Studies*, vol. 9, 2014, pp. 127-145.

"I Am Siri, Award-Winning Porn Star, 2013 Top Writer on *Quora*, and Swinger. AMA!" *Reddit*, 6 Jan. 2014, www.reddit.com/r/IAmA/comments/1ui9v9/iam_siri_awardwinning_porn_star_2013_top_writer/. Accessed 26 Feb. 2019.

Johnston-Robledo, Ingrid, and Joan C. Chrisler. "The Menstrual Mark: Menstruation as Social Stigma." *Sex Roles*, vol. 68, 2013, pp. 9-18.

"Join." *BloodyTrixie*, www.bloodytrixie.com/join.html. Accessed 26 Feb. 2019.

Kipnis, Laura. *Bound and Gagged: Pornography and the Politics of Fantasy in America*. Duke University Press, 1999.

Kristeva, Julia. *The Powers of Horror: An Essay on Abjection*. Columbia University Press, 1982.

Krzywinska, Tanya. "The Dynamics of Squirting: Female Ejaculation and Lactation in Hardcore Film." *Unruly Pleasures: The Cult Film and its Critics*, edited by Xavier Mendik and Graeme Harper, FAB Press, 2000, pp. 31-45.

Lawson, Caitlin E. "Pixels, Porn, and Private Selves: Intimacy and Authenticity in the Celebrity Nude Photo Hack." *Celebrity Studies*, vol. 6, no.4, 2015, pp. 607-609.

Moore, Lisa Jean. *Sperm Counts: Overcome by Man's Most Precious Fluid*. New York University Press, 2007.

Paasonen, Susanna. *Carnal Resonance: Affect and Online Pornography*. MIT, 2011.

Saunders, Rebecca Inez. "The Pornographic Paratexts of Pornhub." *Examining Paratextual Theory and Its Applications in Digital Culture*, edited by Nadine Desrochers and Daniel Apollon, IGI Global, 2014, pp. 235-251.

Seale, Cassie. "This Is Why We Should Embrace Period Sex." *The Nerve*, www.nerve.com/sex-2/this-is-why-we-should-embrace-period-sex. Accessed 7 Aug. 2016.

Sexual Encounter Group. Directed by Alex DeRenzy, Vinegar Syndrome, 2017.

"She's Definitely a Big Deal." *Christian Sings the Blues*, 12 July 2008, cwians.typepad.com/christian_sings_the_blues/2008/07/she-is-definite.html. Accessed 24 Feb. 2019.

"Stoya Episode, The." *Guys We Fucked*, 16 Nov. 2010, soundcloud.com/guyswefucked/stoya. Accessed 4 Mar. 2019.

Williams, Linda. *Hard Core: Power, Pleasure, and the Frenzy of the Visible*. University of California Press, 1999.

Williams, Linda. "Porn Studies: Proliferating Pornographies On/Scene: An Introduction." *Porn Studies*, edited by Linda Williams, Duke University Press, 2005, pp. 1-23.

Ziehm, Howard, et al. Audio Commentary. *Star Virgin*. Directed by Howard Ziehm. Vinegar Syndrome, 2016.

Chapter Four

"Changing the Conversation" about Menstruation from "Very Personally Yours" to #ItsNotMyPeriod: A Discursive Analysis of Menstrual Products and Advertisements

Cayo Gamber

This chapter interrogates a series of distinct texts that purposefully discuss menstruation. Each text is analyzed in terms of the conversation it initiates about menstruation and menstrual products. In particular, this chapter analyzes textual moments and spaces over five decades, in which the conversations around girls' and women's menses were markedly altered. This discursive analysis is based on one of the most cited metaphors in philosophy, literature, and writing studies. It is a metaphor that addresses not only the ongoing nature of conversation but also the nature of critical inquiry, the construction of arguments, the way we conduct research, how ideas unfold, and the academic enterprise itself; it is a metaphor that has alternately been referred to as the unending, ongoing, or interminable conversation—or Burke's Parlor. Kenneth Burke asked interlocutors to envision the following:

Imagine that you enter a parlor. You come late. When you arrive, others have long preceded you, and they are engaged in a heated discussion, a discussion too heated for them to pause and tell you exactly what it is about. In fact, the discussion had already begun long before any of them got there, so that no one present is qualified to retrace for you all the steps that had gone before. You listen for a while, until you decide that you have caught the tenor of the argument; then you put in your oar. Someone answers; you answer him; another comes to your defense; another aligns himself against you, to either the embarrassment or gratification of your opponent, depending upon the quality of your ally's assistance. However, the discussion is interminable. The hour grows late, you must depart. And you do depart, with the discussion still vigorously in progress. (110-111)

This chapter examines how I entered into conversation about menstruation and then looks at ongoing efforts on the parts of those who produce menstrual supplies and those who market them to influence the ways in which we speak—or fail to speak—about our menstruating bodies.

I first learned about menstruation one day when I was in fifth grade[1] during a unique session at the American School[2] in the Philippines. That day, in 1965, my class was divided by gender. The boys went to the gym where they discussed puberty for a short while and then played capture the flag. The girls went to the theatre where we watched *The Story of Menstruation* (1946). The film explained the advent of menstruation and "was framed by a narrative of a pubescent girl's happy daydreams of going on dates, having a wedding, and caring for a baby, the life trajectory that menarche was supposed to set in motion" (Freidenfelds 53). The protagonist of this story, as Sharra Vostral aptly notes, was "a girl with a large head and puny body much like the Tinkerbell character from Walt Disney's *Peter Pan*" (123). The film was one of Kimberly-Clark's most successful educational initiatives; along with other educational materials, it was distributed, for free, to schools around the world. The ten-minute animated film, produced by Walt Disney in 1946, was used in classrooms for over thirty-five years and was viewed by more than 105 million girls (Vostral 121-122).

However, it was not the film but the educational pamphlet—which reproduced the film in written form—that I remember most vividly.

In fact, according to Lara Freidenfelds, "among the most important sources of information about menstruation were the pamphlets created by menstrual product manufacturers, especially Kimberly-Clark" (48). Education pamphlets, such as the one I received, were widely circulated[3] because, as Freidenfelds explains, these pamphlets purposefully separated menstrual education from sex education:

> During its first twenty-five years of creating pamphlets, Kimberly-Clark's commissioned authors managed to write booklets for girls which provided enough information about menstruation to seem useful to parents and daughters but not so much detail about sex or reproduction that parents were reluctant to share them.... Parents were much more willing to educate their daughters early about menstruation if they could avoid talking about sex, so for many girls, the availability of these pamphlets made the difference between having some explanation of menstruation and receiving no information at all. (25)

Jane Ussher also takes note of the emphasis on menstruation itself rather than on sex or reproduction. She argues that education at school "invariably focuses on menarche as a biological event, with girls' interpretation of this important stage in sexual development negated or ignored, and thus concealment is the predominant concern in young women's accounts of menstruation" (20). Here, Ussher is addressing the fact that girls learn to conceal the fact that their bodies menstruate. However, during my introduction to menstruation, concealment was discussed in a different, more literal fashion.

On that day in 1965, at the conclusion of the movie, when we each received our copy of the pamphlet *Very Personally Yours*, we were warned that the boys would be curious about our booklets. We were told boys were not to be allowed to see them. Boys, it was suggested, should not be part of our "very personal" introduction to menarche. This warning recalls David Linton's apt argument that "women [and I would add, girls] have been conditioned to view their periods as private matters whose existence must be kept as closely guarded secrets. But, of course, secrets are not simply kept, they are kept from someone else. And that someone else is the ubiquitous, unnamed male presence" (99-100). Perhaps it is because I was warned to guard my pamphlet that it has become the most marked memory of that particular day.

Now, fifty-three years later, I still clearly remember the cover of the booklet. It was reminiscent of those Victorian cards, where a Caucasian, well-manicured hand is depicted reaching across the card to hand the recipient a rose. However, on this booklet, the hand was holding an invitation that said *Very Personally Yours.*

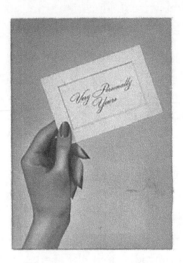

Copyright Kimberly-Clark Worldwide, Inc. Reprinted with Permission

We were invited to read this pamphlet, created by Kimberly-Clark, which promised it would provide us with the information we needed in order to learn to smile through "certain" days. Inside the booklet was a hand-drawn figure of the large-headed perky, white, blonde-haired girl from the movie who smiled as she showered and smiled as she went cycling during those certain days.

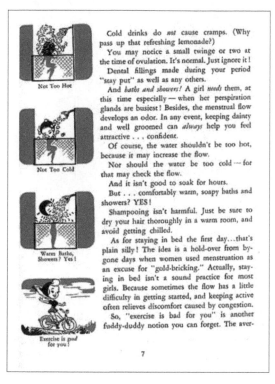

Cold drinks do *not* cause cramps. (Why pass up that refreshing lemonade?)

You may notice a small twinge or two at the time of ovulation. It's normal. Just ignore it!

Dental fillings made during your period "stay put" as well as any others.

And *baths and showers!* A girl *needs* them, at this time especially — when her perspiration glands are busiest! Besides, the menstrual flow develops an odor. In any event, keeping dainty and well groomed can *always* help you feel attractive . . . confident.

Of course, the water shouldn't be too hot, because it may increase the flow.

Nor should the water be too cold — for that may check the flow.

And it isn't good to soak for hours.

But . . . comfortably warm, soapy baths and showers? YES!

Shampooing isn't harmful. Just be sure to dry your hair thoroughly in a warm room, and avoid getting chilled.

As for staying in bed the first day...that's plain silly! The idea is a hold-over from by-gone days when women used menstruation as an excuse for "gold-bricking." Actually, staying in bed isn't a sound practice for most girls. Because sometimes the flow has a little difficulty in getting started, and keeping active often relieves discomfort caused by congestion.

So, "exercise is bad for you" is another fuddy-duddy notion you can forget. The aver-

7

However, in the text of the booklet, there were some caveats. We were warned that we should be considerate of others and not use a swimming pool during our menstrual cycle. (Swimming in a lake, however, was fine.) We were told that we should shower—especially given that there would be odours to wash away—but we also were warned that we needed to be careful to monitor the temperature of the water. If the water were too hot, we would increase our menstrual flow; if it were too cold, we would stop the flow. At the end of the booklet, we were reassured that all would be well during our cycle if we used the Kimberly-Clark products advertised within the booklet.[4]

When I went online to see if I could find a facsimile of the booklet I was given, I realized just how marked a memory I had of this event, for I recalled the booklet in near-perfect detail.[5] I also was chagrined to learn that the booklet we were given was the 1948 version, not the more-timely 1961 version with its "mod" cover.

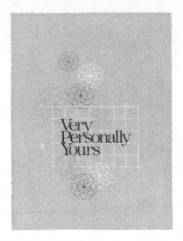

Mindy Erchull, Joan C. Chrisler, Jennifer A. Gorman, and Ingrid Johnston-Robledo note that when girls are questioned about what they have learned about the actual biology involved in menstruation, the girls' answers are vague or inaccurate.[6] I am similar to those girls. I recall very little about the way in which the physiology of the menstrual cycle was described. Although I have a marked memory of the cover and the girl smiling as she showered and cycled, when I try to recall the inner workings of a woman's body, I recoil at trying to really remember what was in the booklet. I know there were anatomical drawings and technical medical language to describe menses; however, my only memory of them is that they made me uncomfortable. It was not because, as Erchull, et al. point out, that the organs oddly floated in space or were inaccurately drawn in terms of scale. I would not have recognized either imprecision.

I think I was like many young girls; I simply recoiled from the images themselves. I was uncomfortable seeing a woman's body anatomically autopsied in this way. In the initial pages of the booklet, the images are of a woman's womb cut in half lengthwise and splayed out on the page. There was one image I recall that made me particularly uncomfortable because the image of eggs in her body reminded me of a jar of Russian caviar. I cringed at the unwitting comparison of a woman's reproduction to that of a fish, and I flinched at the thought of her eggs being bottled as the fish eggs were.

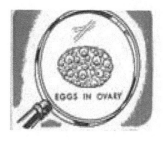

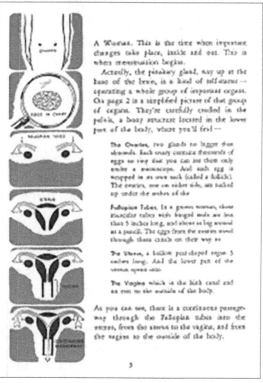

This memory also is revealing in terms of the way that this conversation about menstruation was being constructed. On the one hand, we were offered a scientific explanation of what was going on. Menstruation is, we were told, a natural process. On the other hand, we also were told that we were supposed to keep menstruation a secret. The stipulation to keep our menses secret was emphasized in both the film we watched and the booklet we received. To accomplish this task, we were instructed to put a placid smile on our faces so as not to reveal what was going on, internally, in our bodies. Moreover, not only did our teachers tell us that we were supposed to keep our knowledge of menstruation secret from the boys, but we were also warned that the boys would try to pry this secret knowledge from us. Finally, we were informed it was our menstrual supplies—from Kimberly-Clark—if used correctly (that admonition is always important to remember) that would protect our secret as well.

As Dacia Charlesworth contends, the way in which we were being educated about menstruation created a "linguistic paradox." We were being told that "the menstrual cycle is natural and normal"—so natural and normal that it appeared to me comparable to that of fish— yet we were being encouraged "to keep menstruation a secret" (Charlesworth 14). Such a paradox leads one to ask that if it were so natural and normal, then why was it necessary to hide the fact that one was menstruating?

In the years that followed my introduction to menses, menstruation was more openly discussed, particularly in the world of teen girl magazines via full-page, carefully constructed advertisements. Although the conversation about menstruation—and, more specifically, menstrual products—was more open in the five decades that followed, the linguistic paradox continued: what was natural and normal,[7] and, perhaps, now no longer so secret still needed to be kept hidden. We were admonished by advertisers and product design that we should never be discovered as a woman who bleeds. As a result, for many of us, our initial uneasy attitudes around menstruation were replaced with a real concern, a fear, about being discovered menstruating.

Whereas my fear in fifth grade was that I would inappropriately share secret knowledge with a fifth-grade boy, now the fear was altered from boys learning about menstruation to actually being discovered as a menstruant. Similar to other girls and women, secrecy, shame, and embarrassment became the primary, primal response to the onset of my cycle. Advertisers told us, again and again, that menstrual supplies would give us security and would give us peace of mind. However, this protection and peace of mind came at a price. As we bought into those notions of "feminine protection," we were also buying into notions of shame about the body, as women were being represented as sullied when menstruating.

In her study of feminine hygiene products advertised in *Seventeen* and *Teen* magazines, between the years 1987 and 1997, Debra Merskin found that "advertisements for feminine hygiene products [were] evolving" (955). In particular, she discovered that the copy of most advertisements worked to dispel specific "fears and concerns" (953) by directly addressing girls' "fears of others finding out that they're menstruating" or "the fear of losing one's virginity by inserting a tampon" (953). She concedes that "the primary texts focus on fear and uncertainty," but she notes that especially in the copy accompanying the advertisements, "they also appear to be working to ameliorate these very natural feelings" (953-954).

This type of evolution has continued. In an effort to more openly communicate with their consumers and more consciously address girls' and women's menstrual inconveniences, in 2000, Kimberly-Clark offered a succinct response to menstruation: **Kotex:** . With their product name followed by a piece of punctuation, the "Red Dot" campaign informed women that "having your period is a fact of life; it shouldn't stop you from living it. Kotex® pads, tampons and pantiliners come in all shapes and sizes, so you're covered no matter the situation. No bulging, bunching or shifting, no embarrassing moments ... just you living your life as if it were any other time of the month" ("Kotex Brand Launches"). Although the Kotex advertisements affirmed menstruation as a biological imperative, they also capitalized on reminding girls and women they should be discreet about menstruation interrupting their lives. Even though periods come at the end of sentences, we were told, our periods[8] interrupt the pro·m, vaca·tion, hot·date, con·cert, sch·ool, ni·ght, and g·ym. In order to be discreet, women were advised to buy an array of products. This advertising campaign playfully played on the use of the punctuation point, the "period"; in the vernacular for menstruation, one's "period"; and, at various points, emphatically declare in specific advertisements—"some things are better left unsaid, 'period.'" According to Allison Fass, "the casual frankness of the Kotex campaign [was] indicative of a new tone in ads for such products, moving beyond shots of women climbing mountains in white pants or demonstrations of blue liquid being poured onto pads." Although the campaign was launched in 2000, the Red Dot was most prevalent in 2004 and 2005: "[the] evolved campaign [ran] a 360 degree communication. The effort include[d] product and packaging innovations; a campaign of print and television; and high impact alternative media choices" ("Kotex Brand Launches"). During this campaign cycle, Red Dot advertisements ran in *Cosmopolitan, Glamor, Seventeen,* and *Teen People*; Red Dot commercials also ran during popular series, including *Dawson's Creek, Days of Our Lives, Felicity,* and *Passions* (Fass).

Commercially available and disposable menstrual supplies have been available since the 1890s when Johnson & Johnson sold, but did not vigorously market, Lister's Towels. In the years that have followed, the product lines and vocabulary surrounding menstrual supplies have exploded, from sanitary pads and belts to a long list of beltless feminine napkins, including the following: pads with two adhesive strips; pads with wings; pads with Tiny Totes for discreet disposal; contoured pads; pads of different sizes, teen regular, long, extra-long, overnight; and pads that are ultra-thin or dri-weave or that offer LeakGuard, Odor-Lock, Xtra Protection, or Clean Scent. There are pantiliners that come in thin, thong, and long. There are tampons with cardboard, plastic, or extendable applicators or digital, applicator-free tampons; there are tampons with different absorbency and sizes: junior, light, regular, super, or ultra. And there are tampons that are scented or unscented, bleached or unbleached. In part, this explosion of products is due to incessant capitalist marketing efforts. Elizabeth Kissling observes that "because capitalist systems require that needs change in order for the system to thrive, the frequent small changes in the products are promoted as accommodations to women's changing needs" (17). Similarly, Chris Bobel claims that "product innovation is admittedly ambiguous. At times the emphasis is more on repackaging than on offering new product functionality" (108). For those who produce and market disposable menstrual products, each change to the product line and attendant marketing efforts calls consumers to attend to the buying choices they are making: "In the United States, four players dominate the FemCare market: Procter & Gamble (P&G), makers of Tampax and Always; Kimberly-Clark (K-C), makers of Kotex and Poise (the latter is a product for incontinence); Johnson & Johnson (J&J), makers of OB and Stayfree; and Playtex Products, makers of Playtex" (Bobel 107). It also is worth noting the Big Four, as Bobel refers to them, often make changes concurrently not only to attract new consumers but also to encourage long-time consumers to maintain brand loyalty.[9]

In addition to all of the mass-marketed disposable products, there also are alternative products to consider. These products, developed for those concerned about the environment or concerned about costs, include cloth menstrual pads, menstrual cups, padded period panties, and sea sponges, all of which can be washed and reused.

And it should be noted that there are those who forego products altogether by promoting free bleeding—the practice of menstruating without using products to absorb or collect one's menstrual flow. As Jen Bell explains:

> More than just a period practice, free bleeding is a movement focusing on people's right to menstruate openly and without shame ... there's nothing unhealthy or medically hazardous about free bleeding, so if you prefer to bleed openly, go for it. But more than just a personal preference, free bleeding can be seen as a call to action for us to openly discuss menstruation, challenge stigma, and consider the health and environmental impacts of our menstrual products. Everyone deserves access to their menstrual products of choice—or to forgo them, if they prefer.

Currently, free bleeding may be the most radical of responses not only to the environmental pollution associated with single-use menstrual products but also to the secrecy surrounding the fecund female body.[10]

Neither Kimberly-Clark nor the other the other three Big Four companies have invested in developing reusable products or in endorsing free bleeding. That said, in 2010, in an effort to solidify its consumer base, Kimberly-Clark vowed to change the conversation around girls' and women's menses. As Andrew Meurer, vice president of the North American group brands of feminine, adult, and senior Care at Kimberly-Clark, explained,

> For the past 50 years, advertisers—Kotex included—have been perpetuating this cultural stigma by emphasizing that the best menstrual period is one that is ignored. The way the Kotex brand will be positioned in the future will be very different. We are changing our brand equity to stand for truth, transparency and progressive vagina care. Moving forward, the tone of the Kotex brand's marketing will adhere to its new tagline—Break the Cycle. ("Kimberly-Clark Introduces")

Given that such widespread academic attention has been focused on "critiques of advertisements for menstruation management products" in an effort "to counteract negative attitudes about menstruation among young girls" (Wister et al. 22), the self-awareness expressed by Meurer and the promise to stand for truth, transparency, and progressive vagina care was laudable and auspicious.

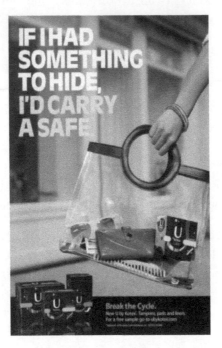

Copyright Kimberly-Clark Worldwide, Inc. Reprinted with Permission

During this last decade, the Break the Cycle campaign has actively combated the long-standing notions of silence and shame that were encoded for so many years in menstrual advertisements. In this particular Break the Cycle advertisement, (see figure above), the box of tampons is prominently displayed in a see-through purse because the woman who carries it no longer needs to hide the fact that not only does she menstruate but that she could be menstruating now. The see-through purse reifies Andrew Muerer's promise to stand for transparency. Girls and women are encouraged to make menstruation real by confronting the subject openly through their own public display of boldly packaged products, such as U by Kotex's black boxes emblazoned with bold colours.

In her research of representations of and conversations about menstruation in the United States from 1870 to 1980, Vostral reveals that "menstrual hygiene products can be interpreted as technologies of passing" (3). That is to say, the products and technologies help to hide the dysfunctional body of the menstruating female and to pass as healthy; these products and technologies "allow women to present themselves as non-menstruants" (Vostral 3). At the conclusion of her in-depth study, Vostral argues the following:

> The examination of menstrual hygiene technologies provides an example of technologies of passing and is one means to discuss how managing the female body and performing termporarily as a non-menstruant reveal deeply embedded assumptions about women's identity in the United States. By recognizing the embedded politics in menstrual technologies, we may begin to challenge them as artifacts of control and instead use them as empowering tools of change. (172)

The Break the Cycle campaign initiates the challenge Vostral calls for.

In addition to print advertisements and television commercials, more recently, Kimberly-Clark has employed multiple online resources as a means of ensuring the menstruant is made visible and the stigma attached to the menstruating body is questioned, derided, and, to varying degrees, dismantled. For example, in a wry series of social experiment videos on YouTube, an actor is positioned in a situation that calls for passers-by to come to his/her help in resolving a menstrual dilemma. In one such video, *Buy Me Tampons* (2010), a young, white, attractive woman stands outside a drugstore on a street in New York. One by one, she asks a series of men who pass by if they could help her out—"I don't have a lock for my bike, and I was wondering if you could just run in and buy me some tampons." In *Help Me Choose* (2010), a young, white, attractive man stands in a store aisle filled with menstrual products; unable to use the word "period" or "products," he turns to a series of men and women who are passing by to ask them to explain what the different products are as he tries to determine which items he should buy for his girlfriend who is on her "___" (the passerby needs to fill in the answer), who asked him to get her some "things."

In each social experiment, the actor engages in conversation with a series of real people. The men who are shown responding to the female actor who does not want to leave her bike unattended are markedly reluctant to buy her tampons. Of the dozen men she engages, one offers to watch her bike and another offers to buy her toilet paper, but none want to engage in a discussion about which tampons to buy and/ or to engage in the actual purchasing of the product. Each time she is turned down she challenges the man with a look of befuddlement or surprise, or she tries to get them to laugh at their own sense of reluctance or revulsion. "You can't say tampons!" she exclaims while laughing. "Every day is about overcoming a fear, right?," she attempts to cajole one man, adding, "So maybe today is tampon day!" The one-minute-fourteen-second video concludes with her calling out to everyone in the street: "Hey, they're just tampons."

In her interviews with women who discussed their lives as menstruants in the 1960s and 1970s, Freidenfelds learned that "interviewees recalled that in the 1960s and 1970s, it was not unheard of for a wife to send her husband to buy menstrual products" (141). A husband "did not expect it to be a regular part of his shopping, but it did not surprise him that his wife would ask him to do this" (Freidenfelds 141). Forty years later, thus, one may imagine that the men approached in *Buy Me Tampons* would be more comfortable purchasing menstrual supplies. In this particular situation, however, it could be that men who might be comfortable buying a product for a wife or partner are markedly less so for a stranger. Moreover, as the *Help Me Choose* video makes clear, these men also may have been fearful about personally choosing among many or trying to find a prescribed menstrual product.

The majority of the men and women who respond to the actor buying products for his girlfriend are remarkably generous in terms of trying to explain a given product or why there would be scented tampons or pearls depicted on one of the boxes for a particular product.[11] During the two-minute-seven-second video, the actor asks over a dozen different shoppers multiple questions regarding the products, including, "what does this mean: regular, super-plus, super?"; "what does that mean—that it's like bigger, like she's heavier set?"; what do the scented ones smell like?"; "what is the necklace for?"; and "do they make ones for runners?" In the end, one woman informs him that given the products he has chosen, he now has his girlfriend covered 24/7 with a product for overnight, for jogging, and for going to work—"ding, ding, ding," she says as she ticks off the three types of products he has chosen and applauds him for covering all his girlfriend's product needs.

These videos make a marked contribution to the menstrual transaction. In his study on men in menstrual product advertising, Linton has lamented that "given that all men and women involved in intimate heterosexual relations must develop ways of dealing with one another in the presence of the period,... it is striking that so little research [and, I would add, so little advertising] has been done on the nature of the menstrual transaction" (112). These videos offer a pronounced effort to change gender attitudes and to change "how men and women [relate] to each other in the presence of the period" (Linton 113). Kissling claims that "menstruation is both a biological event and a cultural event"; moreover, she observes that "how a society deals with menstruation may reveal a great deal about how that society views women" (*Capitalizing* 2). In these social experiments, we are offered a view of how some members of society deal with menstruation, and we can see evidence that men and women are beginning to work towards what Kissling calls "menstrual justice"—"menstrual justice will mean that menstruation is no longer each woman's shameful secret, but a fact of life that need not be concealed" (*Capitalizing* 126). "Hey, they're just tampons," after all.

The most recent Kimberly-Clark campaign has made use of all forms of social media to reach out to millennials. On the U by Kotex website, in the information and advice section, a visitor has written the following two-fold question: "why is menstruation deemed 'gross' and 'disgusting'? [and] why is something that is natural and healthy looked down upon?" Each question is answered from three perspectives— that of a peer, a mom, and a health expert. This question, which received 1781 "likes," received the following responses:

PEER ANSWER[12]

Amazing question. I want to say, "Because some people are idiots," but that'd be mean and honestly, I'm not really sure of the answer myself. Why is something so natural looked down upon? Or worse, made fun of and made into a joke? No idea.

Completely baffling, right? You'd think that because half of the world's population goes through it, it'd be less taboo. Unfortunately not. I think that the problem is that even women and girls look down on menstruation. There are girls and women out there who are embarrassed of their periods. This, I think, sets us back in our movement to show people that periods are neither the warning signs of an apocalypse or reenactment of *The Exorcist*, but rather, that they're simply periods. It's hard to show boys and men that periods aren't something shameful when there are girls and women out there who aren't able to embrace that fact themselves. This is what this campaign is all about. It's so awesome of you to see your period for what it is, natural and healthy, and for what it's not: gross and disgusting.

MOM ANSWER

What a great question. Unfortunately, there's no great answer.... In ancient times, menstruating women were even thought to be possessed by the devil. Sounds crazy, right? I think it was just a lack of understanding then and there's still a lack of understanding today. Many people think a period is something that needs to be hidden and that we need to be "protected" and "kept clean." All of those things can lead to girls feeling ashamed of something that's perfectly natural. If all of us that view menstruation as something that's natural and healthy keep talking about it, hopefully society will eventually become more comfortable with it.

EXPERT ANSWER

This is a great question! Throughout history, women's periods have been considered "taboo": something that must be kept hidden from others because is it unclean and shameful. Though our knowledge of why menstruation occurs has progressed, and we now understand that it is a critical component of women's reproductive cycles, these old attitudes are hard to change. Perhaps nowhere is this as evident as it is in advertising for "feminine products" such as pads and tampons; which cannot even use the words "menstruation," "blood," or "vagina!"

Many girls are creating new dialogues about menstruation and women's bodies. They are speaking out against these old-fashioned practices, and sharing a sense of pride in their bodies with others. You don't have to write a blog or a newspaper column to speak out, though. Sometimes being a role model for other girls, particularly those who are younger than you, can be a very powerful agent of change. So, the next time you find yourself feeling ashamed of your period, or see a ridiculous ad on TV, think of it as an opportunity to create a new conversation about periods. Who knows? Perhaps the next generation of girls and women will laugh when they hear about how "old fashioned" we were when it came to talking about a normal, healthy part of the female experience. (U by Kotex)

The language of the responses echoes the words of the "declaration of real talk" that visitors to the site are asked to sign. Those who sign the declaration pledge to talk openly, to celebrate their bodies, to respect their vaginas, and to challenge society. Conversation and education are seen as the primary ways of changing how girls, boys, men, and women regard menstruation and the menstruating body. There are similarities and differences in how the respondents articulate their answers. All three respondents echo one another as they affirm what a good question the visitor has asked. In addition, they all affirm the visitor that she is quite right: menses is normal, natural, and healthy. However, there are some differences among the three. The peer's voice—punctuated by her use of "that'd," "you'd," and "it'd"—is meant to be colloquial and friendly. (Although the use of the word "apocalypse" does not register as a word a peer would use, and the reference to *The Exorcist* is markedly dated.) The mother's voice is meant to be comforting: all we need is more understanding and menstruation no longer will be seen as gross and disgusting. And, finally, the expert's voice is marked by the challenge she offers the visitor by calling for her to become an agent for change. As the differences among the responses make clear, there clearly is something scripted about these responses as they create a carefully tiered reply, moving from friendly to comforting to inspiring.

In the #ItsNotMyPeriod Campaign, U by Kotex has taken a riskier, more revolutionary approach to changing the conversation. If you have not seen the video *Your Period Doesn't Define You*, it would be worth it to stop reading now, watch the video, and then come back to this chapter because this video challenges all of us to confront how we view women. In *Your Period Doesn't Define You*, approximately a dozen people are invited to watch a quick scene of the inner office workings of a team of four people (three women and one man). The scene in the office depicts a stressful moment at work. One woman who takes charge of the situation speaks more loudly than the others, and then she gives them orders about what needs to be done. Each of the office workers agrees to take on a specific task and the meeting comes to a close.[13] When the viewers are asked, "from that scene, who do you think is on her period?" all of the viewers choose the woman who was, in their words, "bossy," "agitated," and "bitchy" because she raised her voice to get everyone to focus on the task at hand. (As will become clear, it also is lovely that the words she raises her voice to say are, "Well, stop assuming.") And then the interviewer flips the script when she asks them three follow-up questions: "who do you think was the leader?" "who would you want on your team?"; and "do you think she's acting like that because she's on her period, or that's just her personality?" All of the viewers agree that they want the bossy, agitated, bitch on their team and are taken aback by the earlier assumptions they made about the woman they had perceived as menstruating.

In three minutes, this scenario helps to dispel notions that a woman's behaviours, moods, and thoughts are influenced by whether or not she is on her period. In three minutes, both male and female viewers are asked to reconsider what it means to witness a woman who is in control and is taking control. Moreover, and most importantly, a product is not offered as the answer (much less three products— something for nightime, something for jogging, and something for work). Here, the answer is about engaging in a conversation where "you listen for a while, until you decide that you have caught the tenor of the argument; then you put in your oar; someone answers; you answer him; another comes to your defense; another aligns himself against you." And then, perhaps, you rethink, put your oar back in and start the conversation again with new discoveries that allow you to interrogate long-held assumptions and to hear the women who raise their voices in order to be heard and to take charge.

In addition to calling for education and honest conversation, advocacy also has become a pronounced way of changing the conversation around menstruation. U by Kotex created a pop-up shop—The Period Shop—in New York that offered women multiple products with which to pamper themselves while menstruating: comfortable clothes, chocolates, and feminine hygiene products. Dedicated to "encouraging space to have an open dialogue about menstruation, U by Kotex said the shop was 'proof that change can be made about the way people think about, talk about, and shop for periods'" (WITW Staff). All of the profits from sales at the shop were donated to Susan's Place, which "provides homeless women with housing support and a safe, supportive environment" (WITW Staff). In a similar, out-reach effort, U by Kotex partnered with DoSomething in order to sponsor a nationwide drive to encourage donations of menstrual products to girls and women in homeless shelters.

Although these efforts are laudable in terms of their desire to create social change, they also are driven by the desire to create brand fidelity. Advertisers strive to create cradle-to-grave loyalty with consumers; here, the desire is to create puberty-to-grave[14] brand loyalty. Also, it is worth noting, that these efforts target millennials in order to capture their allegiance early. DoSomething, for example, is an organization for young people interested in social change and boasts 5.5 million members in 131 countries. Though driven, in part, by profits, there still is a great deal to be said about the conversation Kimberly-Clark is promoting today. Instead of informing young girls that in order to be considerate of others they should refrain from using a swimming pool while menstruating, young women are called upon to be considerate of homeless girls and women by donating products that will help provide for their needs and dignity.[15]

As a close analysis of these texts reveals, the discourse around menstruation has been changing. Rather than referring to menstruation as a monthly crisis and calling for secrecy and discretion, today the conversations around menstruation humorously, creatively, and deftly address the need to speak openly about girls' and women's menstrual cycles, to dispel the notion that women behave differently when menstruating, and to find inventive solutions to the social and health issues that menstruating girls (and women) confront nationally and globally. What all of these texts share is the desire to ensure that the menstruating body remains visible by making it natural and necessary to talk about bodies that menstruate and by making sure that this discussion combats stigma, promotes menstrual health, and stays "vigorously in progress." It is a conversation with which we can engage—with honesty, humour, and passion—in parlours and in homes as well as in schools, homeless shelters, drugstores, supermarket aisles, and pop-up stores, and among girls, women, boys, and men at the national and international level.

Acknowledgments

I would like to thank students in my Introduction to Women's, Gender, and Sexuality Studies course who, over the years, have joined me in interrogating the way that the marketing of menstrual products complicates and/or informs our understandings of menses. As always, I am grateful to the members of my writing group—Sandie Friedman, Phyllis Ryder, and Christy Zink—who commented on an earlier draft of this essay. I am thankful for Berkeley Kaite's insightful and generous editing of this piece; she consistently asked me to reobserve my observations and astutely pointed out ways for me to refine my analysis. Finally, thank you to the Kimberly-Clark Corporation for allowing me to use the images I have included in this chapter.

Endnotes

1. The timing of when I saw the film confirms Lara Freidenfelds's findings that:

   > Initial advertising for the film did not specify for what age group it was meant, though it quoted happy teachers who had shown it to seventh and eighth graders. The teaching guide that could be requested to accompany it encouraged teachers to address menstruation informally with fourth graders and then show the film in seventh grade. According to a 1964 memo from Kimberly-Clark's educational department, teachers quickly began showing the film to younger students in the fifth and sixth grade. (54)

2. In later years, the school would be renamed the International School.

3. The success of these pamphlets is evidenced by the fact that by 1964, *Very Personally Yours*, written for seventh and eighth graders, and *You're a Young Lady Now*, written for fifth graders, "had together been distributed to about 31 million girls" (Freidenfelds 56).

4. "Kimberly-Clark's pamphlets reached so many girls because they were distributed in a multitude of ways. Unlike other sex education materials, which were primarily available through schools and in some libraries, these pamphlets [also] were advertised widely and could be obtained for free by mailing in the coupons included at the bottom of many Kotex advertisements" (Freidenfelds 46).

5. Erchull, et al., astutely observe that

> Many girls read and reread those little booklets to find out what menstruation is, how they might feel when they experience it, when it will happen, and what to do when menstruation does occur. Although the booklets might not be as common or as important as other sources of information (e.g., mothers, girlfriends, magazines, health education classes; Koff & Rierdan, 1995b), they are a source that is remembered vividly by many women as part of their pubertal experiences. (456)

6. Erchull, et al., cite E. Koff and J. Rierdan's study of 224 sixth-grade girls in which they "found that participants had only the most basic understanding of the menstrual cycle and reported a great deal of misinformation. When questioned about the cause of menstruation, only 3 [out of 224] respondents knew that menstruation occurs when the lining of the uterus is shed because fertilization did not occur" (457).

In their own examination of twenty-eight educational booklets that covered a sixty-five year span (1932-1997), Erchull, et al., found that:

> Later booklets did not have significantly fewer anatomical inconsistencies than did the earlier booklets. A few of the booklets failed to show any of the external genitalia.... The diagrams of the female reproductive organs that are separate from any bodily reference present a particular problem, as it is impossible for a girl to imagine the scale of her reproductive system if she is not given a body outline

to help her understand where the organs are located. How accurate could girls' perceptions of their bodies be if these booklets are a major source of information? (469-470)

7. As this chapter will make clear, these two words, "natural" and "normal," along with the word, "healthy," have become three of the most used and well-intentioned words in communication about the menstrual cycle.

8. I would add, that in her analysis of then-current menstrual products, Berkeley Kaite aptly observed the word "blood" never appears. In addition, Elizabeth Kissling notes that while the word "period" has only been used in recent years, references to blood have remained verboten. As she explains, the language and images related to menarche are "highly circumscribed" (Kissling, "On the Rag" 5). Many scholars have noted that when fluid is shown—for example, when advertisers wanted to show how well a given product works to protect against leaks—there was a tendency to use blue water as a substitute for red fluid. The Red Dot Campaign, thus, while calling for secrecy, also demonstrated a desire to more openly represent menstrual fluid.

9. There always has been an intriguing irony when it comes to what those in the industry of feminine care products have desired in terms of product visibility and the message of their marketing campaigns that promised invisibility:

> Feminist scholars have pointed out, rightly, that menstrual products manufacturers have contributed greatly, through their advertising and other practices, to the sense in American culture that menstruation is embarrassing and must be kept hidden. It is true that manufacturers aimed most of their product development at creating products that hid menstruation as thoroughly as possible, and then, in touting those benefits of the products, promoted the idea that menstruation should be kept secret. However, manufacturers were not necessarily pleased at the direction their industry took. It was difficult to promote and sell products that people were embarrassed to be seen buying and that retailers were uncomfortable promoting locally. (Freidenfelds 137)

In fact, as Thomas Heinrich and Bob Batchelor clarify, as a result of women's reluctance to speak to drugstore employees and pharmacists—many of whom were male—in the 1920s, Kimberly-Clark invested in a "multimillion-dollar Kotex marketing campaign" designed to establish "brand-name recognition through advertising, enabling customers to ask clerks for sanitary napkins by demanding the neutral sounding Kotex—and without having to utter the dreaded term [i.e., sanitary napkin]" (49).

10. Members of the Big Four companies have made changes to address concerns about the environment—including, modifying the packaging in order to use fewer resources (e.g., less plastic wrapping), promoting cardboard applicators rather than plastic, or eschewing applicators altogether. However, given that they are disposable products used over many years of a woman's life, menstrual products are a burden on the environment:

> It is estimated that approximately 20 billion pads, tampons and applicators are being sent to North American landfills annually. On an individual level, each of the approximately 73 million menstruating people in North America will throw away 125 to 150 kg of disposable menstrual products (or 16,800 disposable pads or tampons) in their lifetime. These products require hundreds of years to biodegrade, particularly if wrapped in the plastic packaging commonly provided for this purpose. ("Environment")

11. Here Kimberly-Clark is mocking a rival brand's Pearl Tampons. The Tampax Pearl campaign, which launched in 2002, highlighted the introduction of a smooth plastic applicator with a rounded tip. In addition to an applicator that was supposed to ease the insertion of the tampon, the product line included images of strands of pearls or a single pearl on packages and in marketing campaigns. On the one hand, the pearls are probably meant to represent the feminine and the proper—a well-presented debutante, if you will. On the other hand, the choice of a pearl is curious given that the genesis of a pearl comes from an irritation or an irritant. Natural pearls form when an irritant, such as a parasite, invades an oyster, clam, or mussel. In order to neutralize the irritant, the mollusk produces fluid, called nacre. The nacre repeatedly coats the irritant, in

concentric layers, until a pearl is formed. The pearl in this marketing campaign, thus, functions as a suppressed and/or suggestive reference to menstrual cramps and menstrual blood—both of which can be read as irritants that invade girls' and women's bodies, repeatedly, over many months and years.

12. Given the use of the term "peer," I imagine we are to assume that the interlocutor is a girl given that this individual is seeking an answer from the U by Kotex website. However, it is possible that the individual is a boy. That said, the choice to employ this particular triad—a peer, mom, and expert—to respond seems more likely if the queries come from young girls. Margaret Stubbs observes that "it is obvious that Internet sites have become an important location for discussions of menstruation and that girls themselves are acting more as their own sources of information" (62). In this case, then, the Kimberly-Clark peer conjoins both the use of online sites and the fact that girls are becoming their own sources of information as they share their growing knowledge and expertise as menstruants.

13. And in a pointed turnabout, the lone male worker declares, "I'll get some coffee."

14. One might expect that I would say menopause; however, as an alternative to adult diapers, Kimberly-Clark also makes disposable underwear and undergarments for people with urinary or fecal incontinence. Thus, girls and women could remain loyal customers for the majority of their lives.

15. I have focused in this piece on girls and women who, for the most part it is assumed, not only can purchase menstrual supplies but also can find safe and hygienic resources when menstruating. Worldwide, the lack of running water and the lack of toilets have been a problem for pubescent schoolgirls. In addition, schoolgirls also are burdened by the expense of reliable, leak-proof menstrual products. The growing awareness of the problem has prompted a recent flurry of nonprofit and for-profit companies to develop low-cost alternatives. For instance, in rural India, women's self-help groups are buying semi-automated machines that provide them with the means to make 200 to 250 pads a day. In Rwanda, a company called Sustainable Health Enterprises (or SHE) is training women to make pads out of banana trunk fibers. In Uganda, a

company called AFRIpads has produced enough washable, reusable pads for 500,000 girls across Africa. These are just a few of the efforts made to provide for pubescent girls globally. (See: AFRIpads—A Monthly Challenge, A Sustainable Solution, Afripads.com; Aizenman, Nurith. "People Are Finally Talking About the Thing Nobody Wants to Talk About." *All Things Considered*, 16 June 2015; SHE: Sustainable Health Enterprises, sheinnovates.com/our-work/; Venema, Vibeke. "The Indian Sanitary Pad Revolutionary." *BBC World Service*, 4 March 2014.)

Works Cited

AFRIpads. "A Monthly Challenge, A Sustainable Solution," AFRIpads, 2016, vrouwenvannu.nl/system/files.../afripads_foundation_annual_report_2016.pdf. Accessed 8 Mar. 2019.

Aizenman, Nurith. "People Are Finally Talking About the Thing Nobody Wants to Talk About." *All Things Considered*, 16 June 2015, www.npr.org/sections/goatsandsoda/2015/06/16/414724767/people-are-finally-talking-about-the-thing-nobody-wants-to-talk-about. Accessed 8 Mar. 2019.

Bell, Jen. "What's All the Fuss about Free Bleeding, and Why Does It Matter?" *Clue.* 19 Oct. 2017, helloclue.com/articles/culture/whats-all-fuss-about-free-bleeding-why-does-it-matter. Accessed 20 September 2018.

Bobel, Chris. *New Blood: Third-Wave Feminism and the Politics of Menstruation.* Rutgers University Press, 2010.

Burke, Kenneth. *The Philosophy of Literary Form: Studies in Symbolic Action.* 3rd edition. University of California Press, 1973.

Buy Me Tampons (2010). *YouTube,* uploaded by U by Kotex, www.youtube.com/watch?v=0S9gC4Nk5Ys. Accessed 8 Mar. 2019.

Charlesworth, Dacia. "Paradoxical Constructions of Self: Educating Young Women about Menstruation." *Women and Language,* vol. 24, no. 2, 2001, pp. 13-20.

"Environment." *Luna Pads,* lunapads.com/pages/environment. Accessed 13 October 2018.

Erchull, Mindy J., et al. "Education and Advertising: A Content Analysis of Commercially Produced Booklets about Menstruation." *Journal of Early Adolescence*, vol. 22, no. 4, 2002, pp. 455-74.

Fass, Allison. "A New Campaign for Kotex Aims to Send a Message to Women Worldwide." *The New York Times*, 10 Oct. 2000, www.nytimes.com/2000/10/10/business/media-business-advertising-new-campaign-for-kotex-aims-send-message-women.html?mcubz=2. Accessed 20 Dec. 2016.

Freidenfelds, Lara. *The Modern Period: Menstruation in Twentieth-Century America*. Johns Hopkins University Press, 2010.

Heinrich, Thomas, and Batchelor, Bob. *Kotex, Kleenex, Huggies: Kimberly-Clark and the Consumer Revolution in American Business*. Ohio State University Press, 2004.

Help Me Choose (2010). *YouTube*, uploaded by U by Kotex, 10 Mar. 2010, www.youtube.com/watch?v=n09SejxpcFA.

"Kimberly-Clark Introduces U by Kotex Product Line." *Kimberly-Clark*, 16 Mar. 2010, investor.kimberly-clark.com/static-files/316105ed-2a29-4954-b519-64be766f37fd. Accessed 20 Dec. 2016.

Kissling, Elizabeth Arveda. *Capitalizing on the Curse: The Business of Menstruation*. Lynne Rienner Publishers, 2006.

Kissling, Elizabeth Arveda . "On the Rag on Screen: Menarche in Film and Television." *Sex Roles*, vol. 46, no. 1-2, 2002, pp. 5-12.

Koff, Elissa and Jill Rierdan. "Early Adolescent Girls' Understanding of Menstruation." *Women & Health*, vol. 22, no. 4, 1995, pp. 1-19.

"Kotex Brand Launches Evolution of Iconic 'Red Dot' Campaign." *Kimberly-Clark*, 20 Oct. 2004, investor.kimberly-clark.com/releasedetail.cfm?ReleaseID=145567. Accessed 20 Dec. 2016.

Linton, David. "Men in Menstrual Product Advertising—1920-1949." *Women & Health*, vol. 46, no. 1, 2007, pp. 99-114.

Merskin, Debra. "Adolescence, Advertising, and the Ideology of Menstruation." *Sex Roles*, vol. 40, nos. 11/12, 1999, pp. 941-57.

"Our Work." *SHE: Sustainable Health Enterprises*, sheinnovates.com/our-work/. Accessed 8 Mar. 2019.

Stubbs, Margaret. "Cultural Perceptions and Practices around Menarche and Adolescent Menstruation in the United States." *Annals of the New York Academy of Sciences*, vol. 1135, no. 1, June 2008, pp. 58–66.

U by Kotex. "Everything You Need to Know about Periods." *U by Kotex*, www.ubykotex.com/en-ca/periods/body-image/why-is-menstruation-deemed-gross-and-disgusting-why. Accessed 2 Jan. 2017.

Ussher, Jane M. *Managing the Monstrous Feminine: Regulating the Reproductive Body*. Routledge, 2006.

Venema, Vibeke. "The Indian Sanitary Pad Revolutionary." *BBC World Service*, 4 March 2014, www.bbc.com/news/magazine-26260978. Accessed 8 Mar. 2019.

Vostral, Sharra. *Under Wraps: A History of Menstrual Hygiene Technology*. Lexington Books, 2008.

Wister, Joseph, et al. "Mentioning Menstruation: A Stereotype Threat That Diminishes Cognition?" *Sex Roles*, vol. 68, no. 1, 2013, pp. 19-31.

WITW Staff. "Go With the Flow: NYC Period Pop-up Shop Fights Stigma Around Menstruation." *New York Times*, 17 May 2016, nytlive.nytimes.com/womenintheworld/2016/05/17/nyc-period-pop-up-shop-fights-stigma-around-menstruation/. Accessed 22 Dec. 2016.

"Your Period Doesn't Define You." *YouTube,* uploaded by U by Kotex Canada, 15 Aug. 2016, www.youtube.com/watch?v=MHsc7cO92mw. Accessed 8 Mar. 2019.

Chapter Five

The Contemporary Art of Menstruation: Embracing Taboos, Breaking Boundaries, and Making Art

Barbara Kutis

Whether they take photographs of menstrual stains, paint bloody stains on women's clothing, or use the fluid as their medium, women artists in the new millennium have renewed the second-wave feminists' efforts to bring menstruation into the cultural conversation and to normalize women's experiences of their own bodies. By highlighting this subject in their art, these artists contribute to the discourse of menstruation within contemporary culture. In their exploration of the cultural assumptions of women's experience of menstruation, contemporary artists Sarah Maple, Rupi Kaur, and Jen Lewis celebrate the female experience by revealing a subject that has been traditionally concealed and hidden from artistic discourse.

In order to reveal the advancements in menstrual art made by Maple, Kaur, and Lewis, one must first understand the cultural implications of menstruation and art historical precedents in art. Only after examining the historical reference, can one examine the systems of knowledge with which each artist engages. These artists are distinct from their artistic predecessors, as these artists not only engage with feminist ideas regarding menstruation in traditional formats of painting and photography, but they also incorporate strategies of humor (Maple), social media (Kaur), and photo technology (Lewis) to present their ideas regarding menstruation in an expanded audience and, thus, participate in the broader menstrual activist movement.

Cultural Implications of Menstruation

In 1949, Simone de Beauvoir addressed the cultural history of female bleeding in her canonical investigation of the patriarchal structures that oppress women, *The Second Sex*. In it, she recounts that the Anglo-Saxons called menstruation "the curse" (40), which is a term that persists to the present day—becoming the title of a 1976 text on the cultural implications of menstruation (Delaney et al.) as well as a text written in 2000, which has the subtitle *Confronting the Last Taboo, Menstruation* (Houppert). The curse, in ancient Greece, was a time when the monthly bleeding of women was considered to reflect the blood and flesh of an intended child, whereas in reality, the healthy woman's body is continually attempting to gestate. The process of menstruation, as Beauvoir recounts, involves not only the ovaries and uterus but also the whole female organism, as there are reactions between the ovaries and the endocrine system, and thus the nervous system. The signaling of receptors, coupled with the negative societal responses to female bleeding, results in the woman feeling as if her body were an "alienated opaque thing," which marks the female body as other. Beauvoir expands: "It is the prey of a stubborn and foreign life that makes and unmakes a crib in her every month; every month a child is prepared to be born and is aborted in the flow of the crimson tide; woman *is* her body as man *is* his, but her body is something other than her" (41). Thus, the phenomenological experience of bleeding alienates woman from her own body. She lacks control of this flow, and thus becomes an "other" to herself. Reading Beauvoir, however, is not necessary to reveal to women that the physical process of menstruation can psychically shift perceptions of the self and cause shame—this is a reality lived and experienced by many women. This shame and altered self-perception, however, can perhaps explain why the subject of menstruation has remained a lacuna within artistic practice.

The root of this othering begins in adolescence. Beauvoir establishes that a girl is perceived as innocent but becomes "impure the day she might be able to procreate" (167). Similarly, the biblical text Leviticus establishes rules and regulations for menstruating women, as do many other texts. Pliny would write that menstruating women tarnish all things with which they come into contact: crops, gardens, bees; also, wine turns into vinegar, and milk becomes sour (Beauvoir 167-70). In many societies, menstruating women are considered threatening and dangerous and should be avoided by men, as their virility may be diminished (Delaney et al. 7-9). The threatening and subordinate status of the female body and her bodily fluids might have caused both artists and art historians to exclude the subject from their works. Artwork produced by men such as Jackson Pollock was interpreted as ejaculatory creations of virility, whereas women's artwork, such as the paintings by Helen Frankenthaler (who is discussed below), was read as a womanly accident or stain (Saltzman 375).

Although many of these concepts of menstruation continue in contemporary society (the avoidance of intercourse, the hiding of menstrual pads and tampons, limited physical activity), historical accounts do indicate a positive or beneficial perception of menstrual blood. Blood was believed to "cure for leprosy, warts, birthmarks, gout, goiter, hemorrhoids, epilepsy, worms, and headache" as well as to work as a love charm, act as an offering, and ward off demons (Delaney et al. 9). This secondary positive meaning of menstrual fluid is one that has been subsumed in dominant narratives of the feminine experience. It is my intention to suggest that like the curative applications of menstrual blood, the artwork by these contemporary artists is evidence of a shift in contemporary culture, wherein women's experience of menstruation is more readily discussed and accepted due to the rise of social media and widespread critique. The artists featured in this chapter highlight menstruation by exploring the phenom- enological experience and couple it with humour, feelings of alienation, and beauty to establish and celebrate the pluralistic experiences of women who bleed.

As such, these works of menstrual art participate in the broader cultural menstrual activist movement, which aims to show using menstrual fluid as positive, subversive, and, as Marissa Vigneault claims, riotous. In 2015, interest in the politics of female blood was renewed with vigour as the then United States presidential candidate Donald J. Trump, in an interview stated "You could see there was blood coming out of her eyes; blood [was] coming out of her wherever," referring to the presidential debate moderator, Megyn Kelly (Yan). The unnamed "wherever" spurred outrage, political debate, and protests—in all forms, including menstrual art.[1] Although the works examined here were not made in direct response to the Trump statement, his words reiterate that a negativity persists as it pertains to women's bodies and fluids. These works provide an alternative vision.

The Visibility of Menstruation and Art

Since the post-World War II era, the history of women, art, and menstruation has been a fraught one. In the 1940s and 1950s, the New York School artist Helen Frankenthaler developed a new method of painting, which she termed "soak-stain," in which she manipulated her paint so that she could move, push, soak, and stain the pigment onto the unprimed canvas. This practice, which built upon the gestural painting pioneered by Jackson Pollock, would be received by critics as evidence of Frankenthaler's womanliness—and ultimately be correlated to her menstrual bleeding. The critic E.C. Goosen asserted that "Frankenthaler's painting is manifestly that of a woman.... What she made with it was distinctly feminine, the broad, bleeding-edged stain on raw linen" (qtd. in Saltzman 375)—thus, this relegated her innovation to that of an uncontrollable and uncritical mode of painting as a result of the "flushing of an empty womb" (qtd. in Saltzman 376). Moreover, Morris Louis, who adopted Frankenthaler's soak-stain method, was praised for his control, strength, and clarity. Friend and artist Kenneth Noland would refer to Louis's work as "single-shot" images—a description that Lisa Saltzman argues, transforms the "soak-stain method into an enactment of male orgasm, allowing Louis—the painter of veils and florals—to join the ranks of the virile New York School painters" (377). In sum, by evoking the menstrual stain in his criticism, E.C. Goosen reiterates the gender divide within the art world: women's abstractions are seen as defiling bleeds and men's application of the same technique are perceived as pleasurable orgasms. It would not be until 1965 when Shigeko Kubota participated in the Perpetual Fluxfest at Cinametheque in New York that the image of the menstruating woman artist would shift. On 4 July 1965, Kubota upended the notion of men painting with their phalluses by attaching a paintbrush to her underwear, squatting over a bucket of red paint, and painting a large sheet of paper on the floor (Yoshimoto 182). By creating marks that resembled menstrual stains, Kubota performed a "women's action painting," which could not be realized by Frankenthaler. Kubota would not continue such performance-based menstrual work, yet her infamous performance is an important precursor to Judy Chicago's and Carolee Schneemann's inquiry into the menstruating body in the 1970s.[2]

As Cornelia Butler has asserted, in the late 1960s and early 1970s, the feminist movement "fundamentally changed contemporary art practice, critiquing its assumptions and radically altering its structures and methodologies" (15). Feminist politics aimed to dismantle the patriarchal system of society, and feminist art, or art influenced by feminism, is no different. Feminist art, as practiced by Chicago and Schneemann, is diverse in media, which is partly in reaction to the strictures of the formalism of abstract expressionism in the 1940s and 1950s. Art practice expanded to include Fluxus, performance, and concept-based art (or conceptualism)—all of which dematerialized the art object and emphasized the idea or message above all else (Lippard viii).

It is in this artistic frame that the popular discourse on menstruation in the 1970s is applied. In *The Curse: A Cultural History of Menstruation,* Janice Delaney, Mary Jane Lupton, and Emily Toth assert that the mention of menstruation in film, television, and the media became common by the mid-1970s. Insults referencing menstrual pads and tampons were explicit and uncensored by the media: *National Lampoon* included a cartoon in which a Spanish man who serenades a woman on a balcony has a bloody tampon flung at him instead of a rose; and *All in the Family* aired an episode titled "The Battle of the Month" in March 1973, in which the main character Gloria has her period and argues with her mother (151-152). The latter, according to Delaney, Lupton and Toth, "generated more mail than any other episode that season, most of it objecting to mentioning the menses" (151-152). Likewise, a similar explicitness was presented in the visual art of Judy Chicago and Carolee Schneemann in the 1970s. In 1971, Chicago, Miriam Schapiro, and their Feminist Art Program students from the California Institute of the Arts produced *Womanhouse* (1971-72)—a project in which the women transformed a derelict and abandoned house in Hollywood, California, into an installation and performance space for one month (30 January to 28 February 1972).

Among the many rooms and performances, Chicago presented a white-walled bathroom filled with sanitary products on its shelves and an overflowing wastebasket of used Kotex pads. On the floor next to this wastebasket, Schapiro recalls, "lies one tampax, painted red—*one* out of the 10,000 a woman uses in her fertile lifetime" (269). Known as *Menstruation Bathroom* (1972), the contrast between the pristine white walls, the overflowing wastebasket, and the visible bloody tampon, exposes and subverts the menstrual etiquette of concealment and cleanliness—the room is open for all to see in its state of disorder. Art historian Carol Ockman recollects her reaction to seeing this room: "I was shocked and I loved it ... the irony in this piece—pristine and messy—the fact the female body can't be contained" (qtd. in Levin 199). Similarly, in the 1972 documentary film *Womanhouse*, many visitors appear visibly shocked but also incredibly moved; they comment that the issues raised by the project are important to the understanding of women and their lived realities (Demetrakas).

Menstruation Bathroom was one of three bathrooms in *Womanhouse*, but it was the only one that directly confronted the lived experience of the menstrual cycle. Although thousands of people attended this exhibition, it is important to note that the work did not serve to normalize the feminine experience of menstruation, perhaps due to its location within a gendered-female space (Green-Cole) and its temporary existence (The building containing *Womanhouse* was later demolished). *Menstruation Bathroom* was a pivotal reflection on the growing presence of menstrual references within popular culture, but due to its temporary nature, a discussion of the work's historical significance is lacking; both the bathroom and *Womanhouse* as a whole have not received significant critical attention, despite the bathroom's reinstallation in New York City in 1995 and later in Los Angeles (Bobel 47).[3]

In a similar statement about menstruation, Chicago created the photo-lithograph, *Red Flag* (1971, figure 1), which presents a close-up cropped view of a woman removing a blood-soaked tampon from her vagina. This may very well be the first visual image of a woman performing this act, and Chicago noted that many who initially saw the image did not understand what the red object was—some even thought it was a blood-covered penis (Bobel 46). By presenting this

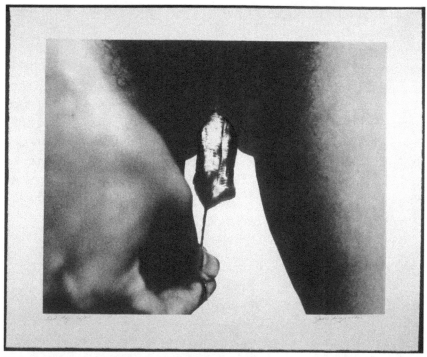

Figure. 1. Judy Chicago, Red Flag, 1971. Photolithograph, 20 x 24 inches. © 2017 Judy Chicago / Artists Rights Society (ARS), New York

vision through the means of photo-lithography, Chicago's image has an element of truth that is bestowed upon the photograph—this is a woman removing her used tampon. It is not an artistic invention, and despite the initial confusion about the work, it is clear that the work is a sort of battle cry for women. By titling the work the idiom, *Red Flag*, Chicago signals that a dangerous menstruating woman is imminent. Yet by calling upon the taboos of menstruation, Chicago asserts the power of women who bleed and suggests that they reveal what they have kept hidden as a means to assert their importance in society. It is through the labour of the woman's body that a new life is born, and, by the same token, menstrual blood is a sign of the life that is not present—and, thereby, the bloody tampon is an item that absorbs the power of life and death, and is located within the woman's body. Through this dual symbolic nature of being both presence and absence of life, the idea of immanence is evoked. Outside the body, the tampon exists as the discarded, the absent. Inside the body, it suggests the vitality of blood and the possibility of life.

Around the same time as Chicago's *Menstruation Bathroom* and *Red Flag*, Carolee Schneemann created *Blood Work Diary* (1972, figure 2), which presents menstrual blood on tissue paper adhered in a grid with egg yolk. Arranged in a grid of four by five tissue squares for a total of five panels, each panel is labelled with the day of the week and time that the sample was collected. Inspired by her former lover's reaction upon seeing menstrual blood during intercourse, the abstract blots challenge taboos and perceptions of the female body. The blots function as indices of Schneemann's body—marking her presence, her absence, and the absence of a child. Yet these blots also appear as a sort of Rorschach test designed to test the subject's perception and personality characteristics.

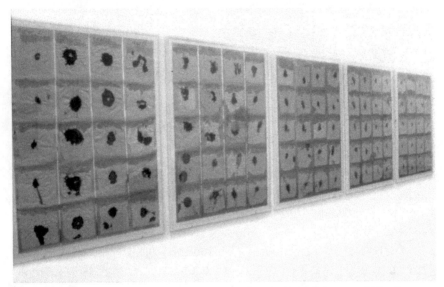

Figure 2. Carolee Schneemann, Blood Work Diary, 1972. Menstrual blottings on tissue, egg yolk, silver paper. 5 panels, 26 x 26 in. each. Courtesy PPOW.

In terms of form, the grid-like repetition of the work engages the conventions and practices of conceptual art, one of the *de rigueur* art forms of American art in the seventies. As *Blood Work Diary* is arranged in a serial and repetitious manner, the designation of the work as a diary places the work within the realm of feminism, as conceptual art is frequently considered an intellectual, esoteric exercise of the male mind. The diaristic, on the other hand, is the personal and feminine, and, thus, inferior. By bringing the biological and the personal into the conceptual practice, Schneemann's work explores the taboo of menstruation and urges the viewer (male or female) not only to reconsider the male dominated traditions of conceptual art but also to reflect upon his or her perception of the natural process and the ways in which women know their bodies (or how men assume women perceive their bodies).

Schneemann and Chicago both explored the feminine experience of bleeding and sought to bring its lived experience to the art world, which had up to that time been predominantly defined as white, male, and heterosexual. Their work was pivotal in the transformation of the art world to a more inclusive space of diverse thoughts and perspectives. By engaging with the cultural taboo of menstruation in the 1970s, Chicago and Schneemann created subversive works that paved the way for future artists' engagement with the issue.

By the 1980s and 1990s, artists such as Kiki Smith, Tracey Emin, and others, would utilize or reference menstruation in their works, yet the menstrual aspect of their works would not be emphasized by the mainstream press. This omission, particularly in the United States, was perhaps due to the "culture wars" that threatened public funding of the arts and was spurred by the photography of Robert Mapplethorpe and Sally Mann. The former featured individuals engaged in sexual homoerotic acts, whereas the later featured the artists own children in the nude. Both projects received criticism from representatives in the federal government and placed the arts, questions of morality, and funding into the national conversation. Similarly, the exhibition *Sensation* spurred controversy in both the United States and in the United Kingdom in the late 1990s. In the US, the exhibition became a subject of national debate in terms of religion—namely because of Chris Ofili's work, *The Holy Virgin Mary* (1996), which featured a dark-skinned Madonna with elephant dung placed at one breast. In the UK, Marcus Harvey's 1995 painting of the child murderer Myra Hindley sparked media outrage and protests because of the work's insensitivity towards the victims' families—the work used children's hand prints to create the visage of Hindley (Becker 15-17). In these particular moments, the inclusion of or reference to menstrual blood in art was not all that shocking or sensational.

How menstrual art became visible in the 2000s was largely due to the rise of social media and fourth-wave feminism. Although third-wave feminists broadened their reach through blogs and e-zines beginning in the late 1990s, it was fourth-wave feminism, which some claim to have begun as early as 2005 (Peay), that utilized social media with aplomb to address issues of sexual harassment, violence against women, and, I argue, menstruation. Fourth-wave feminists capitalized on social platforms to disseminate ideas, to organize, and to contest misogynistic practices (Munro 22). As I argue below, the rise and expansion of social media has allowed for discussions driven by the populous rather than by major media outlets—thus, providing such artists as Maple, Kaur, and Lewis an opportunity to create a conversation around menstruation.

Millennial Approaches to Menstruation

In her essay "Bloody Women Artists," Ruth Green-Cole astutely observes that contemporary women artists who engage with menstruation and blood in their work help to create what she terms "equivocal and polysemous heterotopia[s] for art." By invoking Foucault's notion of heterotopias or sites that "create room for displaced bodies to act" in her examination of artists Tracey Emin, Amy Jenkins, Joana Vasconcelos, and Shilpa Gupta, Green-Cole establishes an important basis through which to examine contemporary menstrual art practices. The artists she examines, as do those I discuss below, explore how traditional structures of power make women feel vulnerable and ashamed, but also open the door to make art that can transform the "stigma and shame into transgressive and creative acts" (Green-Cole) through dissensus.

Sarah Maple (b. 1986) is best known for her humorous works that deal with taboos of Islam at the intersection of Western culture. As a British artist raised as a Muslim (her mother is Iranian Muslim, and her father is an English Christian), much of her work serves as an investigation of her personal struggle as a Muslim living in a predominantly Christian society. In her performance video, *Freedom of Speech* (2013), Maple states:

A lot of people are interested in my work culturally as being brought up as a Muslim and living in a western society, and through the media and how the media represents women in the western world, and so a lot of my work, the process of the work and how I start is I do a lot of reading and research and then I come up with ideas of how I can kind of um expell [sic] my ideas in an accessible way so that I can speak to an audience on a wider level.... And to me that connection with the audience is the most important thing because without that I don't see how they can appreciate the art or take something away from it. And that's why I choose to show my work in humorous ways in um bold ways to kind of grab the viewer's attention. (37)

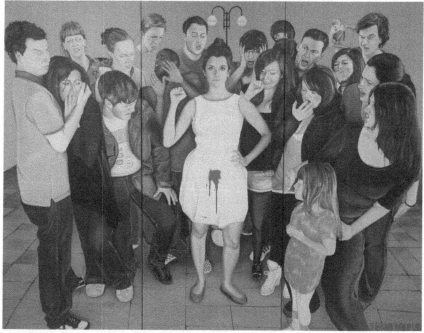

Figure 3. Sarah Maple, Menstruate with Pride, 2010-2011, Oil on canvas, 84.6 x 102.27 inches. Courtesy Sarah Maple.

By using humour to gain the attention of her audience, Maple can transgress social taboos, such as menstruation. In 2010 and 2011, Maple began a large-scale painting titled *Menstruate with Pride* (figure 3), which features a central figure wearing a white blood-stained dress surrounded by nineteen figures (and a monkey) visibly reacting to the presence of a woman bleeding in public. This figure, a self-portrait of

Maple, confronts the viewer with one her hand on her hip and the other raised in a fist of solidarity—as if to visually symbolize the titular rallying call "menstruate with pride!" Akin to Chicago's *Red Flag*, Maple asserts the danger of the woman who bleeds but transforms her person into one who calls for both men and women to see the menstruating woman as a role model of confidence and, perhaps, even power. Unlike Chicago's cropped and fragmented female body, Maple's bleeding subject is fully visible and is shown as a whole person, suggesting an individual with agency. As Maple provides the viewer a clothed woman, standing with a raised fist and confrontational facial expression, Chicago's work provides a view of a woman's pubic hair, thigh, and hand—her identity is reduced to a fragment of her body. Although this representation corresponds to Chicago's ideology of a "'visual symbology' organized around the form of a 'central cavity'" (Chicago qtd. in Meyer 368)—which Chicago (and her colleague Miriam Schapiro) would implement as a means to upend a discourse of sexual degradation—her efforts were largely seen as essentializing and reifying of the male gaze by feminist critics and scholars. The woman is nothing more than her sex, which is to be consumed. Maple's work, however, defies this reading of the female body.

Maple's frank self-possession and pride in her body and bodily fluids are in contrast to the exaggerated grimacing, turning, and visibly repulsed faces of those surrounding her. A man to her right turns and squats down to get a better view of the offending blood; the woman to his right turns her body to the man next to her for protection and solace, but she turns her gaze to Maple to continue to witness the horrific sight. A man immediately behind Maple throws both his hands in the air and turns his head away, as if she and her bloody stain will contaminate his being and, thus, his virility. Others, to the left of Maple, grimace and place their hands near their faces to indicate their shock. Even the small monkey in the background has its mouth agape at the horror of the sight, suggesting that even primates do not approve of such public displays of blood.

Through this painting, Maple conveys the stigma of uncleanliness as well as the concealment required by society of the menstruating body. It is by no accident that she wears white, a colour symbolic of innocence and purity, as she bleeds. Nor is the presence of a young girl to the left of Maple—this is the only figure who does not react in visible disgust or revulsion. This girl gazes intently at Maple's bloodstain, which is at eye level, and displays both hands locked together at her chest. Maple's figure is a role model of what is to come for this young girl. She has not yet experienced the impurity of menstruation, although Maple hints at its impending presence—the pink shirt of the young girl has begun to drip down her white pants.

The feminine associations with blood, as mentioned previously, have traditionally required segregation and subordination—in both the Christian and Muslim contexts. The religious considerations of blood are not lost upon Maple, as both the composition of the painting and the presence of a woman wearing a niqab in the background refer to religion. By creating the painting to appear as if it is a triptych, Maple imbues her scene of menstruation with a religiosity typically reserved for images of Christian saints and holy figures. This quasi-religiosity suggests Maple's work is making a statement akin to Christ's words at the Last Supper: this is my body, and this is my blood (Matthew 25:25). Yet this is blood of a woman; thus, it is an impure bleeding with which others will not make a covenant. To make such a claim could mock the Christian faith, yet Maple claims that mocking is never her intention. She aims to expose the inequities of both blood and faith, and she does so by unilaterally attacking all aspects of it with a sense of irony or humour. As such, she includes a Muslim woman wearing a niqab in the background of her image as well. This Muslim woman bears strong resemblance to Maple herself and, thus, creates a doubling of the artist. Torn between her Muslim upbringing and her Western life that could be said to have opposing cultural views, as Islam maintains tradition and contemporary Western culture allows greater female presence within professional, educational, and social life. Maple's Muslim woman judges the bleeding woman through her enlarged eyes and raised eyebrows—the only part of the body visible of this niqab-wearing woman. The woman's expression evokes the exaggerated actions of silent film comedies of the 1920s, wherein the punchline of a slapstick scene may be deciphered only through the actor's facial expression. Thus, Maple's decision to include the witnesses to the central woman's bleeding creates a sort of comedy stage in which the pride of menstruation can be performed, ridiculed, and tested both by the audience in the painting and the one in the gallery. This is a kind of comedic strategy that is persistent in Maple's oeuvre. On her use of comedy, Maple reveals the following:

> I was always interested in comedy.... I love toilet humour and
> silly things like that, and I approach my work in that way. I
> approach serious things in a really humorous and lighthearted
> way. It's a good way to get the message across, but it has also
> been detrimental. People can think I'm mocking, when this is
> not my aim, that I'm not taking the subject seriously when it's a
> very serious subject. I've approached things in a tongue-in-
> cheek way, and some people can't grasp that. (qtd. in Alice Jones
> 126)

By approaching her work through the lens of humour, Maple
attempts to circumvent social taboos and inner censors, as Sigmund
Freud suggests is the power of comedy. Jokes, as Jacki Willson has
argued, provide a strategy to engage and expose social and moral
judgments (9). By juxtaposing a young girl and a menstruating
woman—a Western woman and a Muslim woman— and by
exaggerating individual reactions, Maple has tuned into a wide range
of cultural implications. Her work clearly rejects the shame of
menstruation in a western context, yet it also engages the strictures of
Islamic tradition. In Islam, it is forbidden for a menstruating woman to
pay obligatory and supererogatory prayers, fast, circumambulate the
Ka'ba, be present in the mosque, and have intercourse. She must
undergo a purification ritual before resuming these activities; thus, to
be seen publicly menstruating would be to flaunt her impurity. This
would be just as sacrilegious as identifying herself as a saint or Christ-
like, so Maple ensures that this scene is ambiguous in terms of how
viewers identify with the work—they may not be amused by such a
display of menstrual pride, and they may not identify with any of the
individual reactions of the crowd that surround her: thus is the nature
of jokes. Freud has argued that the power of jokes lies in the "coupling
of dissimilar things, contrasting ideas, 'sense in nonsense,' the
succession of bewilderment and enlightenment, the bringing forward
of what is hidden, and the peculiar brevity of wit" (14). These are some
of the strategies that Maple utilizes to communicate her subject, and it
is what Beverley Knowles has argued allows Maple to get "at the heart
of the issue, no matter what the issue might be" (9).

Humour is what was lacking from the early feminist works of

Chicago and Schneemann. Their approaches to female bodily fluids aimed to expose the injustices of the female body, but as Amelia Jones recounts in her essay "Sexual Politics: Feminist Strategies, Feminist Conflicts, Feminist Histories" their works were considered to be essentializing by feminist scholars and commentators (409-410). Similarly, the artists in the 1970s lacked the presence of social media to disseminate and spread their work. An article in the British newspaper *The Independent* recounts that Maple had a "faithful following on MySpace before she had a degree" (Alice Jones). This following, in conjunction with the controversial yet comedic nature of her works, boosted her visibility as an artist and continues to act as a platform for her art practice. Similarly, social media is what brought the Canadian poet and artist Rupi Kaur (b. 1992) critical acclaim.

From Painting to Photography and Social Media

Social media has transformed the way in which people communicate, businesses advertise, and artists promote their work. Although many users of sites such as Facebook and Instagram use the platform as a tool to share personal images and thoughts among their friends and followers, the sites also provide a means to engage with the postmodernist tendency of dissensus—that is, a sharing of a plurality of ideas and establishing a discourse of dissenting ideas (Ciszek 316). Moreover, one may consider Jacques Rancière's concept of dissensus in relation to the politics of aesthetics and his notion of a democratic art. Rancière defines dissensus as a "conflict between a sensory presentation and a way of making sense of it, or between several sensory regimes and/or 'bodies'" (*Dissensus* 139). In *The Politics of Aesthetics,* Rancière asserts the idea of a democratic art as the result of emancipation and what he theorizes as the "distribution of the sensible." Emancipation, he argues, occurs when the artist knows that they cannot make others share their views and when the art object "renounces the authority of the imposed message, the target audience, and the univocal mode of explicating the world," or "it stops *wanting* to emancipate us" ("Art of the Possible" 258). For Rancière's notion of the "distribution of the sensible," the distribution of the objects, affects, pleasure, and pains that are apprehended by the senses become structures for how an individual may perceive, think, and act (*Dissensus* 139).

It is in this context that an Instagram post made by Rupi Kaur in March 2015 establishes dissensus. The image assaults the senses through the visibility of the menstruating woman and thereby reframes the social acceptability of menstrual blood within the blurring spheres of social media and art. The potential Instagram viewer must decide whether the post is art (and thus has an intellectual, political, or personal value) or yet another diaristic, self-promotional, or salacious post among the myriad. The power and answer lies within the viewer.

Like Maple's woman in white, Kaur's image features a clothed woman with a menstrual stain on her gray sweatpants. Yet unlike Maple's woman who stands facing the viewer, Kaur's image shows the woman reclining in bed with a mirrored stain on her bedsheets and turned away from the viewer's gaze (figure 4). Thus, the viewer is positioned as an imposing voyeur who stumbles upon the woman's morning discovery of her blood while scrolling through their Instagram feed. The image, intentionally created with a soft focus to alleviate the assault of the subject matter, establishes a private, intimate scene of a woman's experience of her body, thereby reinforcing the sense of secret looking (Kaur, "Period.").

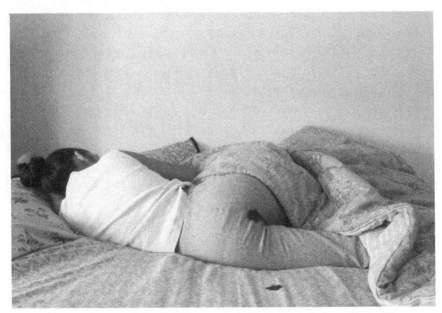

Figure 4. Rupi Kaur and Prabh Saini, period, 2015. Digital photograph. Photo courtesy Rupi Kaur and Prabh Saini.

Part of a series of six photographs titled *period.* (2015), which was created by Kaur with her sister Prabh for a visual rhetoric course, the image challenges the taboo of menstruation, speaks to the artist's own struggle with her monthly cycle, and explores how she could embrace this aspect of her lived experience without using words. The image, initially shared with her then thirty thousand followers on Instagram, was shared with thousands of others within hours. Once the image expanded beyond her initial circle of followers, comments ranged from not understanding why she would post such an image to outright belittlement. Subsequently, Instagram (Kaur, CBC Arts) removed the image. Kaur would then post the image again only to have it removed again. In a third post, Kaur responded to the platform of Instagram as a whole (25 March 2015): "Help keep @instagram safe from periods. Their patriarchy is leaking. Their misogyny is showing. We won't be censored." This post garnered over a thousand comments and generated Instagram's reversal of its censorship. Upon the reinstatement of her photograph, Kaur composed the following message in conjunction with the image. (Note, Kaur uses lowercase letters and periods within her poetry as a reference to the Gurmukhi script used in her native Punjabi tongue. This script is unique as it does not differentiate between uppercase and lowercase—in Kaur's own words, "all letters are treated the same" (qtd in Jain). This is yet another way in which Kaur attempts to disrupt the status quo.)

> thank you @instagram for providing me with the exact response my work was created to critique. you deleted a photo of a woman who is fully covered and menstruating stating that it goes against community guidelines when your guidelines outline that it is nothing but acceptable. the girl is fully clothed. the photo is mine. it is not attacking a certain group. nor is it spam. and because it does not break those guidelines i will repost it again. i will not apologize for not feeding the ego and pride of misogynist society that will have my body in an [sic] underwear but not be okay with a small leak. when your pages are filled with countless photos/accounts where women (so many who are underage) are objectified. pornified. and treated less than human. thank you. (Kaur, *Instagram*)

Kaur's statement reveals the patriarchal and hypocritical system by which society still operates. Although Instagram claims to provide a visual voice for all, it found a fully-clothed woman offensive and in violation of its community guidelines, while as Kaur poignantly states, nearly nude women who are objectified and sexualized are deemed acceptable. The irony of these actions by the company reveal the persistence of the taboo of menstruation within contemporary culture. Instagram's actions caused Kaur to compose the following prose in addition to the *period.* series:

> i bleed each month to help make humankind a possibility. my womb is home to the divine. a source of life for our species. whether i choose to create or not. but very few times is it seen that way. in older civilizations this blood was considered holy. in some it still is. but a majority of people, societies, and communities shun this natural process. some are more comfortable with the pornification of women. the sexualization of women. the violence and degradation of women than this. they cannot be bothered to express their disgust about all that. but will be angered and bothered by this. we menstruate and they see it as dirty. attention seeking. sick. a burden. as if this process is less natural than breathing. as if it is not a bridge between this universe and the last. as if this process is not love. labour. life. selfless and strikingly beautiful. (Kaur, *Instagram*)

These statements gained 91.7 thousand likes and her followers exceeded 600 thousand—near celebrity status (Jain). By using the image and the written word as a mode by which to create dissensus, Kaur escalated a discourse on the normalization of menstruation—not all comments posted on the site are in accordance with Kaur's view, and that is a positive thing. Kaur asserts, "social media is the artist's playground in this post-Internet era. It has become the stage to showcase our work—the gallery space for the common woman and man" (Kaur, *Hunger* 475). By this accord, Kaur's work has the potential to generate a greater impact on the discourse and normalization of menstruation than her feminist predecessors did. What the lasting impact of this work will be is uncertain, but one can hope that works such as these that cross the boundaries of art and social media will continue to establish dissensus.

One can interpret Kaur's image and prose not only as a critique of the exploitation of the female body within social media, but also as a way to promote a discussion on menstruation more broadly—both in the Western and South Asian context. In *Bloody Women Artists,* Green-Cole recounts the strictures on women in India that continue to this day: women are barred from entering some religious temples and monuments while menstruating, and societal taboos "make menstruation unspeakable, not to mention invisible, even amongst women" (Green-Cole). We hear and speak more about the cultures that shun menstruation than we do about those artists who celebrate it and its "selfless and strikingly beautiful" form.

Technology and Beauty

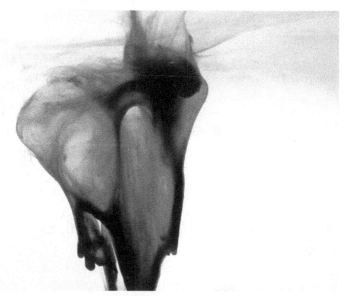

Figure 5. Jen Lewis, Cobra, from Beauty in Blood, 2015, photograph, 24 x 18 inches. Courtesy Jen Lewis.

Unlike the previous two artists who used paint to mimic their references to the menstrual cycle, American artist Jen Lewis (b. 1979) utilizes her own menstrual blood to "challenge the notion that menstruation is 'gross,' 'vulgar,' or 'unrefined'" (qtd. in Hall). As such, Lewis's series of photographs *Beauty in Blood* celebrates the experience of the female form and transforms the pejorative blood into beautiful, ethereal forms that swirl and drift in nebulous shapes (figure 5). Akin to the *Blood Work Diary* by Schneemann, Lewis's images function as indices of her body, but rather than functioning as two-dimensional Rorschach-like blots, the indices are volumetric shapes that dance across the picture plane, sometimes evoking figuration and, at other times, pure abstraction.

Lewis recounts that the stimulus for her series, unlike the impetus for Schneemann's work, was when she "switched from tampons and pads to a menstrual cup at the recommendation of my physician" (qtd. in Frank). She continues: "The cup is a much more 'hands-on' approach to menstruation management so my relationship with my body began changing immediately following the first use. One day, when I had some blood on my fingers after emptying my cup, I started to wonder about why society framed up menstruation as something disgusting" (qtd. in Frank). For Lewis, this change caused menstruation to become something transformative and empowering.

To celebrate the now-changed relationship she had with her own body, Lewis enlisted the assistance of her partner to photograph her blood as she poured and swirled it in the stark white porcelain toilet bowl. Captured with the technology of macrophotography (photographs taken with a powerful camera lens that can magnify the subject tenfold), Lewis is able to capture the unique and abstract forms created by the fluid of her body. She uses a variety of tools to manipulate the fluid as it flows in the porcelain vessel, and like Schneemann's work, records are made of the collection dates, the frequency, and the observations made of each cycle (Lewis). Interestingly, the images themselves are not truly seen until they are seen on the computer—the macro lens of the camera captures shapes and forms not readily visible by the naked eye. Lewis selects images for their aesthetic quality, which suggests there is a beauty contained within the so-called shameful menstrual blood.

As such, Lewis titles the works according to the shapes they imply—for example the blood in *Cobra* evokes the venomous snake that has the ability to rear upward and is known for the hood its skin creates when threatened. *Cobra* mimics the form of the snake through the varying concentrations of blood. The darker, almost black, areas suggest the head and body and the hood through the transparent red and pink on the left. The form that emerges simultaneously appears soft and billowy and harsh and threatening. Paired with the menacing title, Lewis evokes both the negative and positive associations of the menstrual fluid—it is scary but also beautiful and full of potential.

By utilizing digital technology, Lewis's work has reached a broad audience through her personal website, *beautyinblood.com*, as well as through articles featured on *Huffington Post* and feminist websites, such as *Bustle* and *HelloFlo*. Coincidentally, the articles and overall interest in Lewis's photographs are also from 2015, predating Trump's incendiary comment by a few months. By focusing on the fluid rather than the body from which it came, Lewis's images really could come from "wherever," but she insists on linking her abstract shapes to menstrual bleeding. By doing so, perhaps one day, the script could be flipped and a statement such as Trump's could be read as one of power and beauty.

The Politics of Blood

Lewis, like Kaur and Maple, celebrates the female body through its fluids. Together, these artists are but a small sample of contemporary artists who engage with the taboos and perceived boundaries of menstruation in hope of transforming this normal bodily function into something that does not cause women shame. If, as Rancière suggests, art has the power to restructure discourse and affect how an individual perceives the social world, the work of menstruation art will continue to emancipate the subject and individual. The art projects of Lewis, Kaur, and Maple expand upon the goals of the second-wave feminist artists before them to create a discourse on menstruation that exposes, normalizes, and aestheticizes the phenomenological experience of being a woman. Through their work and the menstrual art of other contemporary artists, the expanding discourse on menstruation may cause women to no longer feel alien to their own bodies but rather embrace their menstruating bodies and proudly proclaim: "I am woman, and I bleed."

Endnotes

1. Sarah Levy, an artist based in Portland, Oregon, used her own menstrual blood to create a portrait of Donald J. Trump in response to Trump's comments.

2. In an interview conducted by Miwako Tezuka for the Oral History Archives of Japanese Art, Kubota reveals that her husband Nam June Paik and Fluxus-leader George Maciunas begged her to perform *Vaginia Painting*, but she did not like the ephemeral nature of performance and defined herself as a sculptor at the time. See Transcript, "Oral History Interview with Shigeko Kubota." Interviewed by Miwako Tezuka. Transcribed by Kanaoka Naoko. Translated by Reiko Tomii. *Oral History Archives of Japanese Art,* 11 October 2009. Cited on *Post: Notes on Modern & Contemporary Art Around the Globe,* 2 January 2014. post.at.moma.org/content_ items/344-interview-with-shigeko-kubota. Additionally, while both Kubota and Schneemann were involved in the Fluxus art movement, there is no clear evidence to suggest that Kubota's performance influenced Schneemann or Chicago; rather, her work is an important precedent for the recent artists of whom I am speaking.

3. In 2007, Temma Balducci brought light to the lack of scholarship and interest in *Womanhouse.* For more information, see "Revisiting 'Womanhouse': Welcome to the (Deconstructed) 'Dollhouse.'" *Woman's Art Journal* vol. 27, no. 2 (Fall-Winter 2006), pp. 17-23.

Works Cited

Balducci, Temma. "Revisiting 'Womanhouse': Welcome to the (Deconstructed) 'Dollhouse.'" *Woman's Art Journal* vol. 27, no. 2, Fall-Winter 2006, pp. 17-23.

Beauvoir, Simone de. *The Second Sex.* Introduction by Judith Thurman. Translated by Constance Borde and Sheila Malovany-Chevallier. Vintage, 2011.

Becker, Carol. "The Brooklyn Controversy: A View from the Bridge." *Unsettling "Sensation": Arts-Policy Lessons from the Brooklyn Museum of Art Controversy,* edited by Lawrence Rothfield, Rutgers University Press, 2001, pp. 15-21.

Bobel, Chris. *New Blood: Third-Wave Feminism and the Politics of*

Menstruation. Rutgers University Press, 2010.

Butler, Cornelia. "Art and Feminism: An Ideology of Shifting Criteria." *WACK!: Art and the Feminist Revolution*, edited by Lisa Gabrielle Mark. The MIT Press, 2007, pp. 14-23.

Ciszek, Erica L. "Digital Activism: How Social Media and Dissensus Inform Theory and Practice." *Public Relations Review*, vol. 42, 2016, pp. 314-321.

Delaney, Janice, et al. *The Curse: A Cultural History of Menstruation*. University of Illinois Press, 1988.

Demetrakas, Joanna, director. *Womanhouse*. Women Make Movies, 1972.

Frank, Priscilla. "Artist Explores the Unexpected Beauty of Menstrual Blood Using Macrophotography." *Huffingtonpost.com*, 5 May 2015, www.huffingtonpost.com/2015/05/05/jen-lewis-beauty-in-blood_n_7205908.html. Accessed 28 Feb. 2019.

Freud, Sigmund. *Jokes and their Relation to the Unconscious*. 1905. Translated and edited by James Strachey. W.W. Norton & Company, 1960.

Green-Cole, Ruth. "Bloody Women Artists." *Enjoy: The Occasional Journal*, Love Feminisms, November 2015, enjoy.org.nz/publishing/the-occasional-journal/love-feminisms/text-bloody-women-artists#article. Accessed 28 Feb. 2019.

Hall, Alice. "Menstruation and Art: Fighting the Stigma." *Lyra Magazine*, 2016, www.lyramagazine.co.uk/uncategorized/menstruation-art-fighting-stigma/. Accessed 28 Feb. 2019.

Houppert, Karen. *The Curse: Confronting the Last Taboo, Menstruation*. Farrar, Straus and Giroux, 2000.

Jain, Atisha. "A Poet and Rebel: How Insta-Sensation Rupi Kaur Forced Her Way to Global Fame." *Hindustan Times*, 22 Oct. 2016, www.hindustantimes.com/brunch/a-poet-and-a-rebel-how-insta-sensation-rupi-kaur-forced-her-way-into-the-global-bestseller-lists/story-DCbkk7EBMxrSjdoFsxQmDM.html. Accessed 28 Feb. 2019.

Jones, Alice. "Sarah Maple: 'I'm Not the New Tracey Emin.'" *The Independent*. 27 Jan. 2012, www.independent.co.uk/arts-entertainment/art/features/sarah-maple-im-not-the-new-tracey-emin-6294299.html. Accessed 28 Feb. 2019.

Jones, Amelia. "Sexual Politics: Feminist Strategies, Feminist Conflicts, Feminist Histories." *Sexual Politics: Judy Chicago's Dinner Party in Feminist Art History,* edited by Amelia Jones. University of California Press, 1996, pp. 20-38.

Kaur, Rupi. "Period. Interview with Jana Roose." *Yen Magazine,* no. 77, pp. 54-57.

Kaur, Rupi. "Poet and Artist Rupi Kaur Battled Taboos about Women's Bodies –and Broke the Internet." *CBC Arts,* 29 November 2015. www.cbc.ca/arts/exhibitionists/poet-and-artist-rupi-kaur-battled-taboos-about-women-s-bodies-and-broke-the-internet-1.3326725. Accessed 28 Feb. 2019.

Kaur, Rupi. (@rupikaur_). "thank you @instagram..." *Instagram,* 25 Mar. 2015, www.instagram.com/rupikaur_/. Accessed 28 Feb. 2019.

Kaur, Rupi. "Rupi Kaur." *Hunger Magazine.* Reprinted on www. rupikaur.com/wp-content/uploads/2016/07/Hunger-Magazine. png. Accessed 28 Feb. 2019.

Kubota, Shigeko. "Oral History Interview with Shigeko Kubota." Interviewed by Miwako Tezuka. Transcribed by Kanaoka Naoko. Translated by Reiko Tomii. *Oral History Archives of Japanese Art,* 11 October 2009. Cited on *Post: Notes on Modern & Contemporary Art Around the Globe,* 2 January 2014, https://post.at.moma.org/content_items/344-interview-with-shigeko-kubota. Accessed 6 Mar. 2019

Levin, Gail. *Becoming Judy Chicago.* Harmony Books, 2007.

Lewis, Jen. "Beauty in Blood?" *Feminist & Women's Studies Association (UK & Ireland) Blog.* 25 Sept. 2013, http://fwsablog.org.uk/2013/09/25/beauty-in-blood/. Accessed 28 Feb. 2019.

Lippard, Lucy. *Six Years: The Dematerialization of the Object from 1966 to 1973.* University of California Press, 1973.

Maple, Sarah. *Sarah Maple: You Could Have Done This.* KochxBos Publishers, 2015.

Maple, Sarah, and Anikka Maya Weerasinghe. "Islam Is the New Black: A Conversation with Sarah Maple." *Art Threat,* 24 November 2008, artthreat.net/2008/11/sarah-maple-interview-islam-new-black/. Accessed 28 Feb. 2019.

Meyer, Richard. "Hard Targets, Male Bodies, Feminist Art, and the Force of Censorship in the 1970s." *WACK!: Art and the Feminist Revolution*, edited by Lisa Gabrielle Mark. The MIT Press, 2007, pp. 362-383.

Munro, Ealasaid. "Feminism: A Fourth Wave?" *Political Insight*, vol. 4 no. 2, 2013, pp. 22-25.

Peay, Pythia. "Feminism's Fourth Wave." *Utne Reader*, March/April 2005, www.utne.com/community/feminisms-fourth-wave. Accessed 28 Feb. 2019.

Rancière, Jacques. *Dissensus: On Politics and Aesthetics*. Edited and translated by Steven Corcoran. Continuum, 2010.

Rancière, Jacques. *The Politics of Aesthetics*. Translation and Introduction by Gabriel Rockhill. Continuum, 2004.

Rancière, Jacques, et al. "Art of the Possible." *Artforum International*, vol. 45, no. 7, March 2007, pp. 256-269.

Saltzman, Lisa. "Reconsidering the Stain: On Gender and the Body in Helen Frankenthaler's Painting." *Reclaiming Female Agency: Feminist Art History after Postmodernism*, edited by Mary Garrard and Norma Broude, University of California Press, 2005, pp. 372-383.

Schapiro, Miriam. "The Education of Women as Artists: Project Womanhouse." *Art Journal*, vol. 31, no. 3, 1972, pp. 268-70.

Vigneault, Marissa. "After *Red Flag*—A Consideration of Menstrual Blood as Riot." Women's Bodies: Fluids, Functions, and Fictions. The Legacy of Judy Chicago and Second Wave Feminist Art, Southeast College Art Conference, October 27, 2017, Columbus College of Art & Design, Columbus, OH. Conference Presentation.

Willson, Jackie. "Piss-Takes", Tongue-in-Cheek Humour and Contemporary Feminist Performance Art." *n. paradoxa*, vol. 36, 2015, pp. 5-12.

Yan, Holly. "Donald Trump's 'Blood' Comment About Megyn Kelly Draws Outrage." *CNN*, 8 Aug. 2015, www.cnn.com/2015/08/08/politics/donald-trump-cnn-megyn-kelly-comment/index.html. Accessed 28 Feb. 2019.

Yoshimoto, Midori. *Into Performance: Japanese Women Artists in New York*. Rutgers University Press, 2005.

Chapter Six

Menstruation and Liminality in Ingmar Bergman's *Cries and Whispers*

Peter Ohlin

In Ingmar Bergman's film *Cries and Whispers* (1973), one scene in particular stands out. A mature woman in nineteenth-century dress disrobes in her dressing room in expectation of her husband's arrival to exercise his conjugal rights. She picks up a piece from a broken wine glass and inserts it into her vagina; the pain is visible on her face. She walks with difficulty to the bed, lowers herself into it, and pulls up the covers. When her husband comes in and watches her in bed, she lowers the sheets, moves her hands between her legs, and lifts them covered with blood, smearing her face with it in an almost ritualistic gesture. She licks her lips. Then she laughs. In the context of other references in the film, this seems like a mock menstruation, and what is the significance of that?

This is the context of the scene. On a late-nineteenth-century estate, two sisters have come to be with their younger sister who is dying from cancer of the uterus. The older sister, Karin, and her husband live in a marriage from hell. In a flashback introduced by Bergman himself on the soundtrack, they have dinner together in silence broken only by monosyllabic phrases. The husband wonders since it's late whether they should forego the dessert and the coffee and go directly to bed. Karin's distaste for this prospect is obvious. She fumbles with her wineglass, which breaks and spills the red wine on the tablecloth (a premonition of countless menstrual stains throughout the film). After her husband leaves for the bedroom, she holds a large piece of glass between her fingers and mutters, repeatedly, the phrase, "it's all a tissue of lies." She repeats the phrase in her dressing room. Bergman had initially intended to show the insertion of the glass into the vagina in gruesome clinical detail; he even engaged a "porn queen" who was willing to perform the act but on the day of the shoot failed to appear. (This was in the 1970s, an era marked in Sweden by extraordinary license in the depiction of sex in cinema.) The scene, as it now stands, shows Karin's thighs, seen from above, and her hand with the glass moving it towards the vagina, which is just off screen. She lets go of the glass but continues to push it into her with one finger. Afterwards Bergman realized that the actress Ingrid Thulin "portrayed the mixture of pain and sensual pleasure with such genius"[1] and that no close-up could have been better (*Bilder* 348). Most of these details invite a kind of psychological reading. Karin hurts herself in order to hurt her husband—a not unfamiliar pattern of behaviour in such situations, though a shocking and extreme one.

At the time the film appeared, Joan Mellen criticized the scene for being regressive and exaggerated:

> It is the blood of being a woman drawn with the special perverse satisfaction that comes with a revenge on men. In a scene of gross exaggeration, Bergman has Karin in bed spread her legs exposing the bloody mess to her prissy little husband in his fur-trimmed smoking-jacket. Smearing blood on her face, she proceeds to lick it off as she revels in her own degradation and in the degradation of her sex. But revenge involves only self-mutilation. The fade to red comes this time as a kind of humiliation, one impossible to forget because it is accompanied by the inevitable cries and whispers. (308)

But Karin's action need not necessarily be seen as what Frank Gado calls "Karin's bizarre revenge" (415). Nor is it simply a repressed and self-mutilating demonstration of the repulsiveness of women, as has been suggested. It is, first of all, Karin's act of defiance and revenge against her husband: *So you find women disgusting. If disgust is what you want—here is disgusting.* Thus, it is one particular feature in the war between men and women of the class and repressed character Bergman is portraying, not men and women in general. Second, however,

Karin's smearing of the face to lick her blood is a kind of regressive act—a childlike playing with bodily fluids that breaks civilized conventions. Third, in terms of the colour symbolism, red as the symbol of blood also stands for the whole array of matrilineal symbols; in primitive societies, Karin's action would be contrasted to the white symbolism of men. In terms of Western societies, white symbolism is normally split into white and black: the latter is the male symbol, and the former is the male appropriation of the female (Turner 124). Note, however, that the oppositions frequently function most markedly in societies in which certain sets of social function are performed by members excluded from the lineage that distributes property and political power. Thus, in a matrilineal society, male father-child relationship can serve across clan boundaries to preserve and emphasize social values outside those of political power. When the two systems confront each other, as they do on certain occasions of ritual violation, "once more we meet with the structurally inferior as the morally and ritually superior, and secular weakness as sacred power" (Turner 125). Thus, in a capitalist patriarchal male society, in which men do business in black suits, the women who are structurally inferior may well be morally and ritually superior; their power is sacred power. In the context of the film, what this means is that although the vision of the film may be bleak and women are just as doomed as the men, men, in fact, are more contemptible, more despicable, and more ridiculous; the women are clearly to be pitied and comforted.

But a psychological reading is ultimately difficult, since one can also choose to see the scene as a demonstration of a neurosis—the result of a social world based on the suppression of women in which women are owned and circulated as just another form of property. Or one could read the scene as a demonstration of how some women are both incapable of and unwilling to break out of their condition. Or, indeed, one could also see the scene as a demonstration of the fundamental sickness of women grounded in their womanness—the curse of their gender. All these readings, as well as others, flourish in the voluminous literature about the film (see Steene 297-302).

The question is what does blood perform here? The issue is more fundamental than the psychological interpretations of the characters. For the glass itself—or more correctly, the broken and splintered glass—is directly and intimately associated with the transparency of the medium and its ability to reflect and represent the world. In this case, under the stress of the violence engendered by the central fiction or, for that matter, the audience's participation in that fiction, that ability is severely limited: what we see is no longer a transparent window into the world of the fiction but the mirror of our own fragmented struggle to come to terms with the images of the fiction. The broken glass—the medium that is instrumental in violating patriarchal convention—is thus associated with breaking and fragmenting the narrative medium itself. The broken glass reminds us that what we are seeing is no longer a self-evident transparent window into the world of the fiction. Above all, Karin's act of mutilating herself is then also a refusal to participate in the patriarchal narrative by asserting the existence of a different kind of narrative, which is symbolized by the redness of her blood.

Let us look closely at the scene one more time. Karin is in her dressing room, and she puts her hand with the glass fragment between her legs; as the camera focuses on her face, we see the shine of sweat on her temples. She then gets up and moves to the door. In a long shot, we see her husband look up from the book he is reading. In another long shot, we see Karin slowly walk up to the bed and ease herself into it; the camera now moves close to her face. In a medium shot, the camera frames the end of the bed, as the husband comes close, removes his pince-nez, and observes her; he gradually looks more and more surprised. We then get a close-up of Karin's hands between her legs: the thighs are smeared with red. In a close-up of her face, she then smears the blood right across her mouth, opens her lips, licks them delicately, and laughs. The scene then fades into red.

There are three focal points here: her husband who is looking; what is looked at—the red space between her legs; and she who is looking at the onlooker—the voyeur. In the first shot, the husband is looking at us: we are the vagina. In the second shot, we see the vaginal area, and we become the husband. In the third shot, the tables are turned: we ourselves are being seen, and we become the object of seeing. Here, we may recognize the look of the stripper—observing and challenging the voyeur looking at parts of her body rather than at her. It is then not so much an expression of utter humiliation as it is of one kind of power challenging the power of the voyeur.

Furthermore, a scene like this also cries out for a reading in terms of the gaze. Rosalind Krauss in her book *The Optical Unconscious* provides some trenchant observations on the voyeuristic dynamics of the gaze in the relationship between the work of art and its observers in the context of modernism, specifically the modernism of seeing. She begins by calling attention to Sartre's description of the consciousness of the voyeur at the keyhole leaping out "beyond him toward the still unseen spectacle of lasciviousness" unfolding behind the door, at the same time realizing that "the sound of footsteps announces that the gaze of someone else has taken him both by surprise and from behind" (97). Thus, the voyeur becomes an object for himself—a "carnal being trapped in the searchlight of the Other's gaze ... opaque to his own consciousness, a self that he therefore cannot *know* but only *be*, a self that for that reason is nothing but a pure reference to the Other. And it is a self that is defined by shame" (98). To be discovered at the keyhole, then, she concludes, is "to be discovered as a body; it is to thicken the situation given to consciousness to include the hither space of the door, and to make the viewing body an object for consciousness" (98). Something similar is going on in the scene we have been considering. After the identification with the vagina, and recognition of oneself as a voyeur in the eyes of the other, the darkness of the cinema is a temporary relief. It is temporary because, of course, the shard of glass is itself associated with the rupturing of narrative (the shared cognitive experience); so here, that very violence makes the viewer acutely aware of his own discomfort. In the same way, then, when the glass ruptures the narrative flow (like blood), it also destroys the documentary ambition of the image (since the transparency of the medium has been violated) and reconstitutes it as the carnal embodiment of desire.

Given this context, the role performed by the blood for Karin is that it makes her untouchable, which is exactly what she wants and does not want. She wants to mark her difference from, as well as her separation, from her husband. At the same time, she wants to get closer to and be touched by her sister Maria. Whereas Karin wants to hurt herself and deny her sexuality in order to hurt her husband, Maria plays with her sexuality in various thoughtless forms of betrayal and infidelities. But when her husband tries to commit suicide with a letter opener and asks for her help, she cannot act and simply runs away. Whereas Karin is marked by a heroic self-discipline, willing herself to an all-consuming hatred of her husband, Maria has no discipline whatever. She plays any suitable role at any suitable moment. In contrast to the two sisters, the other two women are outside the influence of menstrual blood: Agnes has lived a virginal life and suffers from cancer of the womb, and Anna has lost her status as mother when her child died. Blood, or the absence of blood, is what permeates all the relationships in the house.

Consider, for example, the physical space the characters inhabit. Every room is dominated by the colour red. The walls are red; most of the furniture is red. In a number of places Bergman comments on this by saying he imagines all that red as the interior of the soul: "When I was a child I saw the soul as a shadowy smoke blue dragon floating like an enormous winged creature, half bird, half fish. But inside the dragon everything was red" (*Bilder* 79). Bergman repeated that description over and over again in countless interviews, probably to deflect questions about what was so important to him about the colour red. In the light of other aspects, such as Agnes's disease (cancer of the uterus) and Karin's self-mutilation, it does not seem too farfetched to see the house itself as an image of the womb. In fact, most of the variations of red on white, or white on red, are related to the appearance of the mother figure: emerging out of a white rosebud, she is wearing a white dress "holding a small, very bright red book" strategically placed in front of her groin (Sitney 47-49). Thus the house can easily be seen as a liminal space, the scene for the passage from life to death. I use the term "liminality" in the sense developed by Victor Turner in a number of his books, which describes the many rituals and sacred spaces connected with the passage from one state to another (e.g., life-death, girl-woman, and citizen-chief). All such passages follow three stages of rituals: separating from the previous life; staying in a marginal liminal world totally different from both the first and the third stage; and entering into the new life or non-life. I do not intend to follow Turner's division slavishly but simply wish to point out that the passage from life to death is surrounded by all kinds of rituals and changes in behaviour. For example, witness the two women who prepare Agnes's body for burial by dressing it in a shroud-like gown and capping her hair with a small neat bonnet. We see only a few little gestures, and then in a slow and measured choreography, the two women make the last adjustments to the body. In a synchronized movement, they open the heavy doors and assume a position on each side of the threshold; they stand there, on guard, as everybody passes in. In the script, all their ritual gestures and actions are meticulously recorded. The passing from life to death is a process surrounded by precise and detailed rituals, the origins and purpose of which may not be immediately obvious.

In fact, this scene has already been predicted at the moment of Agnes's agonizing attack before her death. When she has a brief respite, she is cared for by her two sisters and Anna, who wash her, dress her in a fresh nightgown, comb her hair, give her something to drink, and read to her. Agnes thanks them for their kindness. At that liminal moment, as if in a ritual preparation of the one soon to depart from them, differences, class distinctions, and sibling rivalries disappear.

Thus, I wish to suggest that the most puzzling elements in the film correspond exactly to the betwixt-and-between features of the liminal condition. In order to pass from one state to another, there is always a period in between in which all the regular laws and strictures cease to be operative; nothing is logical, bound by statute, or rational. No established laws apply. It is anti-society and anti-community. It is a space outside of time and narrative. Agnes is dead but not dead. The sisters are alive but muted and paralyzed; they can speak but cannot speak. The film cannot tell us why; it simply demonstrates it. In the liminal state, there is no either/or; everything is both/and. The experience of being suspended between life and death allows for a new liberating insight into otherwise problematic relationships and choices. For example, having recognized that the film is to be about something very simple, a woman who dies, "but gets stuck, as in a nightmare, halfway there and asks for tenderness, to be spared, to be freed" (*Bilder* 86), Bergman meditates on the silent images in his mind of the three women when he records a sudden change: "23 April: Today, on my morning walk, these women started to speak and said clearly that they really wanted to speak as well. That in fact they wanted to have substantial occasions to make themselves understood and that one really can't get at the thing we want to get at without words" (*Bilder* 86). What is remarkable here is that the fiction invades the process of creation, which is supposedly giving it life. This is to transgress all ordinary narrative boundaries. Like Agnes who is dead and not-dead, the women are now both fictional and not-fictional. In this world, this liminal world, it makes little sense to try to determine what is real and what is fictional or what is waking and what is dream. The two worlds merge with each other, as August Strindberg says in the preface to *A Dream Play*: "Everything can happen; everything is possible and likely ... The characters split, double, multiply, evaporate, condense, dissolve and merge. But one consciousness rules them all: the dreamer's; for him there are no secrets, no inconsistencies, no scruples and no laws. He does not judge or acquit, he merely relates" (80).

In one of the best accounts of *Cries and Whispers*, P. Adams Sitney writes:

> The elaborate linkage of gestures, both rhyming and reversing, throughout the film should not surprise us; for here, as often elsewhere in Bergman's work, the different characters of the films are vectors, of a single fantasy system which generates its narrative complexity by scattering and redistributing its aspects among imagined persons who are in essence a single haunting presence. (48)

This is undoubtedly true, but what makes it so haunting is Bergman's understanding that the particular fantasy system would only work within the context of a liminal universe as described by Turner or, for that matter, by Strindberg.

What does all this have to do with the theme of menstruation? The liminal space of the film comes to an end when Agnes dies for the second time, guided by Anna. In the aftermath of her death, Karin and Maria are having a brief discussion about their relationship. Karin is shuffling some papers. Maria asks her what she is looking at. Karin says it is Agnes's diary and reads: "I have received the best gift a human being can ever get in this life. The gift has many names: solidarity, communion, human nearness, tenderness. I think this is what is called grace." In most films, whenever a letter or an extract from a book is read aloud, it is not so much intended for the characters in the film but for the film audience. In this case, this is emphasized by the fact that when Anna, who is in the next room, hears Karin read the words, she looks up, hastens to the door, and remains there, listening with rapt attention. It is a message from beyond the grave, a letter from Agnes. It returns in a slightly different form in the final sequence of the film.

That sequence stands out for several reasons. For one, it is an exterior shot. After all that time in a world which is either white and red or black and red, we are finally given the full spectrum of colour in an autumn scene. It is a transformation of extraordinary power. It is as if a difficult journey has finally reached its goal. Agnes has come to rest. The liminal world, its obliteration of established boundaries and traditional rituals, can now be abandoned. After Agnes's death, life will go on. This is not a rejection of death but an affirmation of simple human experience: "It is not a rebirth, a spring; rather, it is a repetition in a different register of the temporality of the whole film" (Sitney 47):

> I shut my eyes and felt the wind and the sun against my face. All the pain was gone. The people I love the most in all the world were with me. I could hear them talking softly around me, I felt the presence of their bodies, the warmth of their hands. I closed my eyes and closed them again, wanted to hang on to the moment, and thought to myself; this must certainly be happiness. I could not ask for anything better. Now, for a few minutes, I can experience perfection. And I feel deeply grateful for my life, which gives me so much. (*Filmberättelser* 187-188)

This is a translation of the notion of grace that Karin reads earlier into the language of the physical body: nearness, bodies, warmth, hands, and moments. The distance that Agnes talks about in the first flashback as she recalls her mother's all too rare acceptance of her needs is transformed into a celebration of physical nearness and perfection. How is this done?

At a moment in the film when Agnes finds herself unable to remain dead, Bergman does the unthinkable (as he so often does). He addresses the reader directly:

> The only thing I know is that I am driven by a desire to lay bare a condition to create a space in the middle of a chaos of confusion and contradictory impulses, a space where imagination and the desire for form in a mutual effort will crystallize into one component in my sense of life itself: the unreasonable and never stilled desire for communion, the clumsy attempts to abolish distance and isolation. (*Filmberättelser* 180)

Here again, we find the opposition of chaos, confusion, and contradictions, on the one hand, and the desire for communion as well as the abolition of distance and isolation, on the other. This is yet another attempt to demonstrate the erasure of the boundary between the author and his fiction, between logic and emotion, contradiction and form. The liminal world of death-in-life and life-in-death—the blood of menstruation and of violent self-destruction—has altered the relationships of all the characters. The title of the film itself points to this opposition: loud cries heard from afar and quiet whispers heard close by. In the end, the imagination and desire for form in the film lead to the moment where the brutality and force of the menstrual stains—Karin's glass, Maria's husband's suicide attempt, for example—engender a moment of peace, serenity, and fullness.

Endnote

1. All translations are my own.

Works Cited

Bergman, I. *Bilder.* Stockholm, 1990.

Bergman, I. *Filmberättelser* Norstedts,1973.

Krauss, Rosalind. *The Optical Unconscious.* The MIT Press, 1993.

Mellen, Joan. *Women and Their Sexuality in the New Film.* New York, 1974.

Sitney, P. Adam. *The Cinema of Poetry.* Oxford University Press, 2015.

Steene, Birgitta. *Ingmar Bergman: A Reference Guide.* Amsterdam University Press, 2005.

Strindberg, August. *Ett drömspel.* Stockholm: Aldus, 1974.

Turner, Victor. *The Ritual Process: Structure and Anti-Structure.* Cornell University Press, 1969.

Chapter Seven

"The Problem Was That She Was a Girl": The Female Complaint in Alice Munro's Juliet Triptych

Kasia van Schaik

I never read a book in a railway carriage without asking,
Is he a builder? Is she unhappy?
—Virginia Woolf, *The Waves*, 56

It's not the tragedies that kill us, it's the messes.
—Dorothy Parker, 86

Anywhere Elsewhere

One summer, while visiting my hometown, a small mountain-locked settlement in Western Canada, I read an Alice Munro story every day for a month straight. It was a necessity, my only semblance of routine. I read her stories by the lake, on the margin of sand between the shoreline and the industrial train track; I read them on my back, legs crossed, book blocking out the sun like a small square flag. Sometimes a train would rumble past and alert me to my environment, which seemed less real than Munro's black spruce or her "fast-flowing, dark and narrow streams," which coursed through many of her stories, linking them the way rivers connect distant parts of the continent (*Runaway* 52-54).

It was a lonely summer, my summer with Alice Munro. I was irritated by the fact that my old friends now had boyfriends and jobs and no longer made time for me—a precocious humanities student back from her studies out east, eager to show off the new words she'd learned. *Liminal. Mimetic. Anagnorisis.* No one cared. I was, essentially, an Alice Munro character. I read her stories to find myself in them but also to distance myself from the unhappy women I encountered in them. *I would do better.* (Secretly, I knew I would not.)

Years later, I would learn that Munro herself had lived in this very town, surrounded by furs and glacial lakes and annual forest fires. This could well be the landscape that flashes past the train window in many of her travel stories—or escape stories—in which a young woman buys a train ticket and heads west or east, anywhere "elsewhere."

What my education in stories yielded that summer was a profound, multilayered, often contradictory, often circuitous articulation of what I would come to know as the female complaint—that is to say, the critique of the double standards and asymmetrical power relations that shape women's lives. I was learning to put words to the growing frustration that since the age of fifteen had been inherent to my experience of the world. I was beginning to understand that the pain of being female—of having a predetermined narrative thrust on my life—was not personal but rather systemically produced by a culture that denies women agency in public and private spheres. This was what it meant to enter into femaleness: to encounter the contradictions that reveal the ways in which the personal is refracted through the general (*The Female Complaint* vii). I came to realize the difficult feelings that I shared with Munro's female narrators were not simply a consequence of unsettled chemistry; they were not "a problem to be fixed" but rather, as Olivia Laing puts it, "a response to structural injustice" (*The Lonely City* 281). These were political emotions. They defined a public wound. The female complaint, in turn, was a tool of address, an "aesthetic 'witnessing' of injury" ("The Female Complaint" 243).

As instructional as Munro's portrayal of the female dilemma was to me that summer, her depiction of the double standards women face— the experience of being double or being doubled down upon—resists didacticism. There are no resolutions, conclusions, or closures in

Munro, only openings. One of the ways in which her work invokes a structure of openings is through her use of nonlinear narrative forms, what Natalie Foy calls the "weird geometry" of parallel, intersecting, and non-continuous threads, which embodies the feeling of being in a world "too much with us" while, at the same time, puzzling and elusive (153). Critics agree that hers is an art of "accommodating contradictions" (Blodgett 30); her stories refuse to surrender "a clear indisputable, and singular meaning" (MacKendrick 26). In their denial of closure, her stories offer their narrators a self-conscious "parody of resolution" (*Runaway* 149). Like the female complaint, they offer an "aesthetic witnessing" rather than reconciliation for expressions of injury. In these ways, Munro's attunement to form reveals a direct correlation to the themes that she returns to in her work—the existential and emotional importance of narrative in shaping human life, particularly in shaping women's lives (Coleman; Thrusser). It is this link that I am interested in exploring in the following essay, specifically, the ways in which the female complaint—the thematic, textual, and, crucially, the physical embodiment of that complaint in the form of menstruation—inform the narrative structure of Munro's work, and, in extension, how Munro's work reflects the ways in which we use narrative to navigate these impasses in our own lives.

Foregrounding the female complaint as a mode of address provides a useful entry point into thinking about the constraints shaping women's narratives. It opens up a conversation surrounding the ways in which gendered double standards have been naturalized and the critique of women's disenfranchisement trivialized. For one, the term the "female complaint" has long been a euphemism for menstruation and "ailments that afflict women; specifically gynaecological ailments" linking the female body with the genre of complaint itself (OED). According to Sarah Stage in *Female Complaints*, her book on women's medical history, the "female complaint" was the "catchall nineteenth century term for disorders ranging from painful menstruation to prolapsed uterus" (27). Indeed, the eighteenth-century physician Alexander Hamilton's suggested treatment for female complaints included everything from "spare living, with increased exercise, occasional blood-letting" and "frequent gentle purgatives" in the form of "an infusion of bark in lime water" to "occasional opiates" and "the injection, several times a day, of warm milk and water into the passage of the womb" (*The Management of Female Complaints* 39-40). As such, the double entendre of "complaint"—its haphazard annexation of both women's medical disorders and menstruation cycles—not only indicates the ways in which women's bodies and bodily complaints are managed but also signals the banality of female suffering. Women's pain is naturalized by routine; women's grievances are rendered unsightly, purely corporal, and apolitical, in so much that they are considered medical conditions rather than responses to systemic oppression.

Furthermore, the female complaint, when used to describe women's menstrual cycles, turns women's bodies into a metonymy for complaint. In other words, not only does the complaint give a narrative shape to women's experiences of being in the world, it also turns the female body into a complaining body, a body that, by definition, articulates itself as a complaint. As Lauren Berlant suggests, the complaint as a mode of self-expression "is an admission and a recognition both of privilege and powerlessness: it is a powerful record of patriarchal oppression, circumscribed by a knowledge of woman's inevitable delegitimation within the patriarchal public sphere" ("The Female Complaint" 243). Depending on its context, the complaint both expresses and institutes limits to its own effectiveness. It offers an expression of dissent while also acknowledging its concession to a system that largely ignores women's complaints. This is because the genre, the very word "complaint," undermines itself and connotes a trivial or minor expression of dissatisfaction: a nag, a gripe, a whine, or a plea. At the same time, because of its banality, its irritating persistence—its very unexceptionally—the complaint becomes a sly but politically powerful form of protest.

Nevertheless, on the Train, She Was Happy

"Chance," the first story in Alice Munro's Juliet triptych (*Runaway*, 2004), begins with a woman reading on a train. Juliet is reading, but she is also menstruating. Her focus is broken by frequent visits to the train bathroom for "reinforcements." Menstruation, the "bane of her life," is imagined as an intrusion on her intellectual pursuits, the female body drawing attention to itself, making a disturbance ("Chance" 61). Juliet is determined not let her bodily complaints disrupt her reading, her doctoral studies in classics, and even her romantic encounters. Yet I would like to suggest that it is Juliet's resistance to confronting her inconvenient body, as well as her inability to eclipse it, that directs the narrative in the story cycle. Her fraught relationship with the female complaint sets up a structure of concealment and disclosure and gives shape to what Dorothy Parker calls the "messes" of the everyday—the small disappointments, confusions, and seemingly minor grievances, which, in the long run, define a life.

It is significant too that the story cycle, which acts loosely as a bildungsroman, should begin on a train. For Munro, the train, like the book, is represented as a technology of access, linking the passenger, and the reader, to the possible worlds beyond a life circumscribed by gender or class or geography. If the messes or "menses" reveal the ways in which the narrative trajectory is interrupted, the train journey offers us a way of thinking about narrative direction. The train is—to apply the word I had freshly learned that summer by the lake—a liminal space. It is a mobile space; a narrative opening in a life hemmed in by social expectations and familial duty. In this way, the train bares a metonymic relationship to the act of storytelling itself. As Raymond Carver contends, in order for a story to exist, "there has to be tension, a sense that something is imminent, that certain things are in relentless motion"; this is achieved not only by "the way concrete words are linked together to make up the visible action of the story" but also by "the things that are left out, that are implied, the landscape just under the smooth (but sometimes broken and unsettled) surface of things" ("On Writing" 277). This description of storytelling resembles the "relentless" trajectory of the train—its linked carriages, the landscape speeding past, glimpsed in reflection, sometimes remarked upon, sometimes left out.

The train is also a contact zone. That is to say, it sanctions a space of contact between strangers and between lives that once uprooted may feel strange or estranging. For instance, in "To Reach Japan," a short story from Munro's most recent collection, *Dear Life*, the narrator leaves behind a husband in Vancouver and, accompanied by her young daughter, travels to Toronto to reunite with a man she met once at a literary gathering; in the train journey in "Wild Swans," a young woman is touched under her skirt by a older male stranger, an event that produces in her both disgust and sustained erotic curiosity; and in

"Chance," an encounter with a fisherman on the train changes the entire trajectory of the narrator Juliet's life. Though bound to its course, the train becomes associated with a libidinous freedom, an aleatory thrust towards a future unknown, "chanced" at. The train journey, like the road trip, allows the female narrator to shed her habitual life and become, as the narrator in another travel story reflects, a "watcher, not a keeper"—that is, an observer, a collector of experiences, and not a keeper of order, of children, of the home ("Miles City, Montana" 88). Yet as we see in Juliet's case, she cannot escape her body and become purely a "watcher." As the menstruation scene, as well as the encounters with men on the train, reminds us, Juliet's body is an interrupting body as well as an interrupted body. She cannot fully transcend her gender and become a spectator or "watcher" because she is already a spectacle.

Juliet is made to feel her gendered position again when her reading is interrupted by "a trousered leg, moving in," a lonely male traveller who asks her, being an independent traveller as well, if she would like to "chum around" with him during their cross-continental journey ("Chance" 54-57). She extricates herself from the company of the man and climbs to the observation deck where she glimpses "a large wolf crossing the snowy, perfect surface of a small lake" and where she also encounters Eric, the future father of her daughter, although, of course, she does not know this yet (57). The next few events happen in quick succession. The train collides with a body on the tracks (it turns out to be the man whose company Juliet rejected), and Juliet is forced to attend to her period, which threatens to become a visible problem and which, later, will be inexplicably mistaken for the suicide's blood. Juliet contemplates writing to her parents of this accidental substitution, but she considers that "the suicide's smashed body ... would seem, in telling, to be hardly more foul and frightful than her own menstrual blood" (64). This shrinking awareness that her body's rhythms would seem "foul" and "frightful" in "telling" is indicative of the anxiety that will preoccupy Juliet throughout the three connected stories: the fear of not fulfilling her role as wife, a "keeper" of an adulterous man, and the fear of "lacking in motherly inhibitions and propriety and self-control" (*Runaway* 156). Or perhaps this is the anxiety that underpins the guilt of performing her female role too well—of over-loving her daughter and of displaying an excessive attachment to another being—to the point that she loses her. These larger anxieties—Juliet's supposed lack of self-control and fear of being unable to contain her emotions, her partner or child—are made concrete in the train scene through the bodily manifestation of "the female complaint," her menstrual blood. She exemplifies what the ancient Greeks considered to be definitive female qualities: she becomes a "leaky vessel," one whose boundaries are "pliant, porous, mutable" and whose power to control them is "inadequate, her concern for them unreliable" (Carson 133).

As we see on a micro-level in the menstruation scene that sets off the Juliet triptych, this mode of excess and the lack of control or discipline over the porous female body not only dictates the narrative but shapes the way in which Juliet understands her position in the world. Monthly bleeding interferes with Juliet's participation in "important three-hour exams because," she points out, "you couldn't leave the room for reinforcements" ("Chance" 61). This acknowledgment, in itself, reveals a subtle critique of a world not build around women's bodily rhythms. But the theme of overflowing one's boundaries, of lacking self-control or self-containment, of "falling hectically in love" with those alarmed by "ready emotions," persists throughout the story cycle, prompting us to question the role her menstrual blood plays in shaping the narrative (*Runaway* 149). Thus, in response to the pivotal question that this collection of essays asks— what does blood perform?—I argue that not only does the presence of menstrual blood work as a plot device, but it is integral to the theme and form of the story itself. It allows for the narrative to be leaky, messy, and not easily simplified or thematically secured. It brings into focus the act of storytelling itself as an art that inhabits the opening between what is said and what is withheld, what is marked, what is concealed, what is reinforced with silence, and what is spilled.

Tell, Never Tell, Tell Somebody Something

The word "problem" is mentioned twice in "Chance," each time referring to a different register of the female complaint. The first acknowledges a structural complaint fundamental to the experience of being female, or rather, entering into femaleness:

The problem was that she was a girl. If she got married—which might happen ... she would waste all her hard work and [her professors'] and if she did not get married she would probably become bleak and isolated, losing out on promotions to men (who needed them more, as they had to support families). And she would not be able to defend the oddity of her choice of Classics ... Odd choices were simply easier for men, most of whom would find women glad to marry them. Not so the other way around. (53)

Juliet's frank articulation of "the problem" of being female exposes the glass ceiling that limited women's careers and creative aspirations in the 1960s (when the story is set), in 2004 (when the story was published), and which still persist today, fourteen years later. She observes that it is easier to be "odd" as a man—an observation that still bares currency. As we see in *The Lonely City*, Olivia Laing's recent treatise on loneliness and art making, Laing reflects that there comes an age for women when "female aloneness is no longer socially sanctioned and carries with it a persistent whiff of strangeness, deviance and failure" (15); where to be a woman, never mind an artist, is to become in Juliet's words "bleak and isolated." This sentiment also reveals the ways in which intelligence in women is cast in a deviant light. As Juliet acknowledges, for women, intelligence and ambition are "often put in the same category as a limp or an extra thumb" (53); that is to say, they are viewed as an impediment, a curiosity, or an excess. Again, to echo Juliet, not so the other way around.

The second mention of "problem" in the story occurs a few pages later and also has to do with excess—in this case, her menstrual blood. What is particularly interesting about the episode on the train, the scene that sets off the cycle of events that will determine Juliet's life narrative, is the relationship between Juliet's menstrual blood and her writing—specifically, the link between her problem and the anticipated disgust it will evoke in her reader or listener if she dared to tell the story (61). This connection between blood and narration, the way the manifestation of the female complaint determines what is told and what is left out, invites us to consider how the role of menstrual blood in this story not only influences the thematic content—the exploration of the double binds women face—but shapes the narrative organization as well. In her study of bodies as living narrative systems, the poet Erin Moure asks, "so what if the inner narrative comes not from the hands alone or the eyes or the ears but from … that vaginal space in us that is continuous & contiguous with the air & has never been counted as Real but as an empty space, unreadable" (110). It is the tension between this sense of unreadability as well as the denial of readability and the desire to be read that shapes Munro's narrative structure and defines the conditions of suspended agency under which the complaint genre operates.

We see this movement between what is told and what is left unsaid in the scene following the suicide on the train. After Juliet overhears other passengers talking about finding the bathroom "full of blood" (63), she concedes that if she were to tell anyone of the event, "people would think her exceptionally crude and heartless" (64). She resolves to "never tell that to anybody" (64). Yet in the very next sentence we find that she does, in fact, disclose the secret at a later date:

> Never tell that to anybody. (Actually, she did tell it, a few years later, to a woman named Christa, a woman whose name she did not yet know.)
>
> But she wanted very much to tell somebody something. She got out her notebook and on one of its ruled pages began to write a letter to her parents. (64)

This oscillation between modes of telling, partially telling, and withholding—the never tell/tell/tell somebody something—is indicative of the narrative structure of the Juliet story cycle, and, in extension, much of Munro's work. The bracketed acknowledgement "(actually, she did tell it)" captures the way in which small disclosures and small omissions are beaded together throughout the narrative as a modality of storytelling. The paragraph break after the bracketed line and the following admission that she "wanted very much to tell somebody something" work in a similar way—capturing the pause, the attempt to resist the telling, the resistance overruled, which emulates the impulse of the teller. The brackets also contain the sudden dilation of time to "a few years later," and allow for three narrative gestures to simultaneously cohabit the story frame: telling (the reader), not telling (the blood is omitted in the letter), and having told (a future friend and, as it turns out, rival). This produces what Maurice Shadbolt calls the short story's ability to produce a "hallucinatory point in which time past and time future seem to coexist in time present" (qtd. in May 269). This temporary coexistence invites the reader to exercise a negative capability, to hold in her mind multiple time-scapes as well as contradictory impulses and to bear both the weight of secret keeping alongside the pleasure of secret telling. In this way, Munro's narratives inhabit that pocket between sound and silence, a place also occupied by the reader, as the act of reading requires the silent sounding out of words. As such, the narrative form allows for what Viorica Patea calls "both the visible and the invisible, the surface and the inner secret of things" to coexist on the page (17). Blood, in this instance, becomes an embodiment of the open secret; it is both an invisible yet hyper-visible performance of the female complaint. It is the ailment that is concealed, but, at the same time, it becomes the substitute for what is seen.

This narrative technique, made up of unsaids, secrets, and false epiphanies, reveals the self-reflexivity so common to Munro's narrators—and one which Carver claims to be intrinsic to storytelling itself —an investment in the present telling of the story, while at the same time acknowledging that "something is imminent, that certain things are in relentless motion" (50). In this scene on the train, the allusion to Christa, "a woman whose name she did not yet know," invites the reader to inhabit the space of contradiction: to register a name, while registering that the name is not known—essentially, to be told and to be untold. Furthermore, the fact that Juliet finds in Christa a future confidant emphasizes the way in which the shared economy of storytelling and its genres—confessions, complaints, or gossip—are informative, pleasurable, as well as protective gestures between women. This creates what Berlant calls the "intimate public" between women seeking permission to "live small but to feel large"; or, in Juliet's case, particularly, to "live large but want what is normal too; to be critical without detaching from disappointment and dangerous worlds and objects of desire" (3). This shared modes of story making legitimizes storytelling as a means of connection and, perhaps, even emotional contingency between women in an environment where trust between women is continually undermined. We, readers, are drawn into this secret network as well while, at the same time, we are made aware of the insistence that, at its heart, every story is only a partially told story, fragments of a whole only guessed at. This mode of telling reflects a contemporary relativism (Patea 19). As Patea contends, the renouncement of an intact "whole" story expresses "an awareness that, in a fragmented, splintered world, wholeness is no longer possible" (19). This narrative mode also reflects the way in which the accumulation of gendered micro-aggressions, disappointments, and misinterpretations can give shape to an experience of life. Once again it recalls Dorothy Parker's observation that "it's not the tragedies that kill us, it's the messes." Put slightly differently, it is the naturalized injustices and the everyday expressions of misogyny and racism that provide the seeding ground for our larger cultural failures.

We see this theme taken up again in another self-reflexive moment of storytelling on the train directly after Juliet's menstrual blood is confused with the suicide's absent blood. As the passengers stand in the dining cart window craning to get a glimpse of the suicide's body, a mother tries to distract her child from the scene at the window by ordering him to colour in his book, and she then chastises him: "Look at the mess you've made, all over the lines" (62). The train rounds the curve, but we find out that "there was no blood to be seen, on either side of the car" only "a trampled area, a shoveled mound of snow" (62). Not only do these two images, slotted beside each other in this scene of spectatorship, recall Juliet's menstrual blood, which then becomes a substitution for the absence of blood on the tracks, but they also allude to the act of writing itself: what is concealed in the snow bank is revealed instead in the "mess ... all over the lines" of the notebook. Cause and effect are confused; the exceptional (suicide) is confused with the routine (menstruation), death, with the possibility of life. This collapsing of binaries emphasizes the way in which a fantasy of a clean linear narrative is constantly disrupted, fractured, and misinterpreted by life's fatal messes. It becomes a micro-version of what Jhumpa Lahiri refers to as Munro's revolutionary method of turning the "[short story] form on its head," (which prompts the spectators on the train (and the readers of the story) to recognize how experience and its recounting—its jarring revelations, shifting judgments, and provisionality—are never clear or singular (Fiamengo and Lynch 4). Thus, by allowing for what Mark Nunes calls "overflow" and the "denial of a totalizing narrative," the narrative "captures the 'funny jumps' of living: bumps that unsettle the narrative frame" (11). As we see in the train scene, these moments of "overflow" and collision give shape to the narrative and, in Munro's own words, signal "everything that is contradictory and persistent and unaccommodating about life" ("Barton Bus" 128).

A Watcher, Not a Keeper

Could it have been the scene on the train that first compelled Pedro Almodovar to adapt the story cycle for his 2015 film *Julieta*? In an interview, he acknowledged, "For me, the set piece in the train is very important. It's also the part of the film that I've kept most faithful to Munro's texts ... I think that everything that happens in the train is like a fantastic and terrible tale" (53). When questioned about why he did not set the film in Western Canada, he explained "I visited Vancouver, but found the landscape so depressing and the light so oppressive that I couldn't picture myself shooting there" (53). The "depressing" landscape and the "oppressive" light are not the only elements missing from his adaptation. Although he remains loyal to the emotional features of the train scene, even including a surreal image of a Canadian stag galloping across the Spanish landscape in homage to Munro (another hallucinatory moment), Juliet's menstrual blood and the misinterpretation of the menstrual blood for the suicide's blood are omitted. This, at first, may not seem like an important detail. In fact, one could argue that the menstrual blood is made atmospheric and is portrayed in the red silks and red walls of Julieta's home in Madrid. Yet as we see in Munro's story cycle and the elegant counter-point it finds in Almodovar's film, the inclusion/exclusion of the menstrual blood not only changes the course of the narrative and the characters' motivations but also alters the structure of the narrative.

In *Julieta*, the absence of blood alters the narrative trajectory. By creating a clear causal relationship between the events and denying the messiness caused by the inclusion of the menstrual blood, the film dramatically shifts where and on whom the emphasis falls. For instance, in "Chance," the fact that the encounter on the train between Juliet and Eric is left unconsummated because of Juliet's fear that he will discover her blood-soaked pad means that her incentive for visiting Eric in Whale Bay is motivated by an active sexual desire, whereas Almodovar's interpretation, we see a more socially acceptable motivation: the maternal drive to finding the father of her child. Like the narrator in "To Reach Japan," whose liaison with a stranger on the train results in the near loss of her daughter, Juliet is an active agent, compelled by her own self-interest rather than filial obligation. In this way, the inclusion of the blood narrative makes Juliet's motivations more radical (especially for a woman in 1960s Canada) because they are rooted in an assertive and, therefore potentially unsettling, female desire.

Juliet's split allegiance to being a "watcher" and a "keeper" lends the three stories their central tension. It appears that she is punished for daring to pursue a life that exceeds the confines of her gender—by leaving her small Ontario town, pursuing graduate school, and eventually finding a career in journalism. Yet she is also punished for attempting to follow a more conventional route, as she gives up on her academic aspirations in order to live with Eric and raise her daughter, Penelope, who ultimately rejects her. In an unvoiced confession— another instance of the slippage between the said and the unsaid— Juliet concedes that her daughter's desertion is "just a way she has found to manage her life" (*Runaway* 157). She imagines Penelope as the Ethiopian queen's lost child, living among nomadic philosophers and "left with a perverse hankering for a bare, ecstatic life" (152). Yet we learn that secretly Juliet has devised a different ending to the myth, "one that would involve renunciation, and a backward search ... [and] reconciliation, at last, with the erring, repentant, essentially great-hearted queen of Ethiopia" (152). Although Munro denies such a resolution, what Juliet reveals in this self-reflexive passage is an aware-ness of her own act of storytelling and her position as a storyteller. Indeed, Juliet describes the project of the story cycle itself—the backward search through a life in order to find meaning in the events, both mundane and tragic, that gave it form. In the end, hers is the "bare, ecstatic life," surrounded by books whose myths do not match up to the uncertainties of history or to a narrative that has failed its conventional arc and has found no resolution.

As Jonathan Franzen has observed of the contradictions so often faced by Munro's female characters, "simply by trying to survive as a whole and independent person, she has incurred painful losses and dislocations; she has caused harm" (Franzen, *Review*). Yet as Jeff Birkenstein points out, there is an uncomfortable sense, often barely glimpsed beneath the surface of Munro's stories: "that the destruction has already occurred before the stories begin, that an impending explosion is waiting just for a spark" (213). Is it then chance or contingency? Or another way to put it is, is there such a thing as chance in a life that has been predetermined by the problem of being female? How to be both a watcher and a keeper? This is the question that surfaces in Munro's work and speaks to the double standards that women still face—this is, essentially, the contradiction inherent in the female complaint: the insistence that woman and women's lives must be double, both, and neither.

The Juliet stories—much more than Almodovar's film—pry open more cracks than they seal. Whereas the film ends with a potential reunion and reconciliation between Julieta and her estranged daughter, the story offers no such closure. As we have seen, the final story opens into yet another story thread—the legend of the Ethiopian queen and her lost daughter—displacing or even parodying narrative closure and emphasizing the cyclical nature of loss and loss as part of the organic rhythms of the body. In this way, the narrative form doubles back on itself, demonstrating the limitations of narrative completeness, the way in which life sheds life (Thacker 37).

Douglas Glover describes Munro's narrative technique as a composition of "resonating structures," which allow for various parts of the text to "echo off each other"; this self-reflexive and self-refracting structure, in turn, reveals the ways in which "the inner life of a man or a woman is also a text ... at our deepest point this is our experience of experience" (35). Thus, it is through aporia, omission, and elliptical spasms that these inner texts enter into language and are simultaneously blurred by language, capturing the charged incompleteness of experience. Munro's leaky structures, as well as her narrative "overflow" and "funny jumps" (Nunes), allow for action to bleed into retrospection, memory into fantasy, and for the dilated narrative present to include both past discomfort and future complaints. This invites us to think about the narrative frame as a kind of gyre, composed of letters, notebooks, and complaints—a system of tracking memory and experience across the expanse of a life. These stories, these "inner texts," are the residue of a life examined, bringing together the told, the partially told, and the unexplained. They describe the "messes" that Dorothy Parker warns us can kill us if left ignored or silenced.

I am reminded of another set of tracks that appear at the very beginning of the Juliet triptych and predict the "weird geometry" of the story cycle. "There were tracks in the snow, small animal tracks," Juliet observes from the window of the train; "Strings of beads, looping, vanishing" (52). Not only do these small animal tracks foreshadow Juliet's fear of leaving tracks and marking the snow with her menstrual blood, they also replicate the image of the printed page—the scribbled lines of her notebook, the half-concealed truths in her letters, and the silent tracking of the story itself. It is through this tracking that Munro's narratives themselves take shape; in this mode they bleed across time, distance, and memory, linking stories within stories, looping, vanishing.

Works Cited

Berlant, Lauren. *The Female Complaint: The Unfinished Business of Sentimentality in American Culture.* Duke University Press, 2008. Print.

Berlant, Lauren. "The Female Complaint." *Social Text,* no. 19-20, 1988, pp. 237-259.

Birkenstein, Jeff. "The Houses that Munro Built: The Community of *The Love of a Good Woman.*" *Critical Insights, Alice Munro,* edited by Charles E. May, Salem Press, 2013, pp. 213.

Blodgett, E. D. *Alice Munro.* Twayne, 1988, pp. 30.

Carson, Anne. "Dirt and Desire: Essay on the Phenomenology of Female Pollution in Antiquity" *Men in the Off Hours,* Random House, 2000, pp. 133.

Carver, Raymond. "On Writing." *Mississippi Review,* vol. 14, no. 1-2, 1985, pp. 50.

Coleman, Phillip. "Friend of My Youth: Alice Munro and the Power of Narrativity" *Critical Insights, Alice Munro.* Salem Press, 2013, pp. 160-175.

Fiamengo, Janice, and Gerald Lynch. "Introductory" *Alice Munro's Miraculous Art: Critical Essays.* Edited by Janice Fiamengo and Gerald Lynch, University of Ottawa Press, 2017, pp. 4.

Foy, Natalie. "'Darkness Collecting': Reading 'Vandals' as a Coda to *Open Secrets.*" *Rest of the Story: Critical Essays on Alice Munro,* edited by E.C.W. Thacker, ECW Press, 1999, pp. 147-68.

Franzen, Jonathan. "'Runaway': Alice's Wonderland." *The New York Times*, 2004, www.nytimes.com/2004/11/14/books/review/runaway-alices-wonderland.html. Accessed 27 Feb. 2019.

Hamilton, Alexander. *A Treatise of Midwifery Comprehending the Management of Female Complaints and the Treatment of Children in Early Infancy*, J. Murray, 1781, pp. 39-40.

Lahiri, Jhumpa. "Writers on Munro", *The New Yorker*. 10 October 2013. www.newyorker.com/books/page-turner/writers-on-munro. Accessed 27 Feb. 2019.

Laing, Olivia. *The Lonely City: Adventures in the Art of Being Alone*. Picador, 2016, pp. 51-281.

MacKendrick, Louis K. *Probable Fictions: Alice Munro's Narrative Acts*. ECW Press, edited by Louis K. MacKendrick, 1983, pp. 26.

May, Charles E. "Biography of Alice Munro." *Critical Insights, Alice Munro*, edited by Charles E. May, Salem Press, 2013, pp. 3.

Moure, Erin. "Hope Stories," *Sheepish Beauty, Civilian Love*. Vehicle Press, 1992.

Munro, Alice. "Barton Bus." *The Moons of Jupiter*. Macmillan of Canada, 1982.

Munro, Alice. "Miles City, Montana," *The Progress of Love*. McClelland, 1986.

Munro, Alice. *Runaway*. McClelland & Stewart, 2004.

Munro, Alice. "To Reach Japan." *Dear Life: Stories*. McClelland & Stewart, 2012.

Nunes, Mark. "Postmodern 'Piercing': Alice Munro's Contingent Ontologies." *Studies in Short Fiction*, vol. 34, no. 1, 1997, pp. 11-26.

Parker, Dorothy. "Interview with Marion Capron." *The Paris Review: The Art of Fiction*, vol. 13, summer 1956-57, pp. 86.

Patea, Viorica. "The Short Story: An Overview of the History and Evolution of the Genre" *Short Story Theories: A Twenty-first-Century Perspective*, edited by Viorica Patea, Rodopi, 2012, pp. 1-26.

Shadbolt, Maurice. "The Hallucinatory Point." *The New Short Story Theories*, Ohio University Press, 1994, pp. 269.

Stage, Sarah. *Female Complaints: Lydia Pinkham and the Business of Women's Medicine*. W.W. Norton & Company, 1979, pp. 27.

Thrusser, Michael. "Narrative, Memory, and Contingency in Alice Munro's *Runaway.*" *Critical Insights, Alice Munro*, edited by Charles E. May, Salem Press, 2013, pp. 242-259.

Woolf, Virginia. *The Waves.* Hogarth Press, 1933.

Chapter Eight

Orange Is the New Black: Menstruation, Comedy, and the Unruly Feminine

Katerina Symes

In season five of the Netflix original series *Orange Is the New Black* (*OITNB*), a riot erupts at Litchfield penitentiary. Amid the chaos and the blaring sound of the prison's emergency alarm, Gina Murphy (Abigail Savage) pounds on a locked office door and demands correctional officer Joel Luschek (Matt Peters) to let her in. Reluctant to share his hiding spot, Luschek tells Gina to "Go away!" She pauses, frustrated. Unwilling to concede defeat, Gina reaches down into her pants (it appears as if she is searching for something, but it is unclear what), and when her hand re-emerges, she smears menstrual blood over her face. Witnessing this event, a nearby inmate, Blanca Flores (Laura Gómez), responds with a resounding "Ugh! And they call *me* disgusting." Gina rolls her eyes at Blanca and continues pounding on the door; this time, she feigns injury as she hysterically pleads with Luschek for help. Upon seeing Gina's bloodied face, Luschek rushes to her aid. As the office door swings open, Gina drops the act: "Okay, we have to cut the alarm. It's making everyone nuts." A visibly distraught Luschek can only stare at Gina's crimson face: "Are you hurt? Where are you hurt?" Sensing Luschek's distress, Gina reassuringly responds, "Oh. No, I'm fine. It's period blood. Heavy flow." Luschek groans and immediately recoils in disgust.

Luscheck's and Blanca's reactions to Gina's menstrual blood reproduce some of the prevailing cultural assumptions of menstruation as tainting, as polluting, and as a lapse in normative femininity, wherein women's leaky bodies must be appropriately managed and contained (Fahs 157; Johnston-Robledo and Chrisler 9; Chrisler 203; Ussher 1). However, the visible presence of menstrual blood, as well as Gina's comical yet casual indifference to her own menstruating body, not only reflects menstruation's complex negotiation within *OITNB*'s comedic form but also posits alternative accounts of femininity beyond women's concealment and regulation of their bodies. Debuting in July 2013, the Netflix original series *OITNB* was created by television writer and producer Jenji Kohan and is based on Piper Kerman's 2010 memoir *Orange Is the New Black: My Year in a Women's Prison*. The critically acclaimed comedy-drama follows the experiences of a diverse group of women at a minimum-security prison called Litchfield, and it depicts a multiplicity of body types and a range of characters with overlapping gender (e.g., cis, trans, masculine, feminine), sexual (i.e., lesbian, queer, heterosexual), class (e.g., working, upper-middle), and racial and ethnic identities (e.g., African American, Caucasian, Dominican, Puerto Rican). As a series about women inmates, *OITNB* foregrounds menstruation to account for alternative modes of femininity that embrace women's leaky, open, and disruptive bodies. This paper examines how menstruation is negotiated within *OITNB*'s comedic form. As I argue, through comedy, humour, and irony, menstruation and menstrual blood become metaphors for the unruly feminine. Indeed, the women inmates are defiant by virtue of being in prison; however, their humorous repurposing of menstrual products as well as their frank and unfiltered discussions about their periods reveal how they can circumvent the limits of their incarceration within a prison space that contains and regulates their bodies.

Menstruation, Comedy, and Normative Femininity

As a comedy-drama, *OITNB*'s engagement with humour and irony offers a space wherein female bodies can be seen, heard, and performed against the norm—that is, the social and cultural assumptions about how women ought to behave and act. As Linda Mizejewski has noted, "women's comedy has become a primary site in mainstream pop culture where feminism speaks, talks back, and is contested" (6). More generally, humour and comedy are contingent upon the "perception of events or behaviour as unexpected or incongruous" (Johnson 272). Irony emphasizes how women's behaviours and actions depart from social and cultural expectations for feminine comportment, and, in doing so, it highlights the regulatory force of the norm itself. This negotiation of inconsistencies and embracing of ambiguities in women's actions and behaviours, thus, position the comedy genre as an ideal space for women to push boundaries and challenge gender ideologies, since an essential aspect of humour is to call the norm into question (Wagner 36; Walker 71).

Scholars working in this area have noted an incongruous relationship between humour and femininity (Kotthoff 5-6; Walker 79). According to Martha Laurzen, "comedy requires the comic to call attention to one's self, an act denoting a position of authority and superiority typically associated with masculinity" (107). Moreover, Mizejewski identifies a historic binary of "pretty" versus "funny," wherein women comedians can transgress ideal versions of femininity precisely because they are constructed in opposition to "pretty," regardless of their appearance (5). Comedy and humour emphasize women as disruptive figures; their grotesque and parodic excesses enable them to act out and defy social and cultural expectations that stereotype women as unfunny, unintelligent, less assertive, etc. (Rowe 11). Indeed, female comedians—such as Tina Fey, Amy Poehler, Wanda Sykes, Sarah Silverman, Amy Schumer, Samantha Bee, and Leslie Jones—pose wicked and formidable critiques of such stereotypes, but it is through the medium of humour that such critiques are softened, made palatable, and heard. Women's parodic excess within comedic conventions mocks tropes of femininity (i.e., ideologies of true womanhood, such as the perfect wife and mother), as the figure of the unruly woman reimagines how women are constructed as gendered subjects (Rowe 11; Rowe 412-413; Russo 225).

Within OITNB, the women inmates are unruly feminine figures; they are defiant not only by being incarcerated women but also by their seeping, oozing, and menstruating bodies. In contemporary culture, menstruation and menstruating bodies become visible in the margins, if at all, and only when written into a pathologizing narrative in which their presence results from a lapse in feminine decorum. Menstrual leaks are a failure to appropriately manage and contain one's body (Erchull 33; Jackson and Falmagne 390; Johnston-Robledo and Stubbs 10-11; Chrisler 203). The peripheral presence of menstruation and menstruating bodies exists only to mark the constitutive outside between so-called good (which is to say normatively feminine) bodies precisely because menstruation serves as a referent for women's failure to discretely contain and dispose of its excesses (Kissling 482).

OITNB is acutely aware of these pathologizing narratives, as it challenges such images of menstruation and menstruating bodies. The series negotiates menstruation through comedy, humour, and irony, and, in doing so, menstruation performs a kind of metaphoric volatility; women's bodies become referents for a defiant femininity— making visible the extent to which the women inmates are always-already bodies out of bounds, even within a prison space that contains them. Through their menstruating bodies, the women inmates exceed the norms of conventional gender representation; they not only reject the "pollution taboos" (Rowe 410) that urge women to sanitize and deodorize their bodies (which foster shame, silence, and self-loathing), but also transgress the unspoken feminine sanction against "making a spectacle" of themselves (Rowe 414-415). In this vein, *OITNB* continues the work of this ongoing scholarship through positing women's bodily experiences as a source and opportunity for agency (Fingerson 85). As Laura Fingerson suggests, although much of the discourse surrounding menstruation is negative (i.e., worries about leaking, or exaggerated claims regarding the emotional effects of menstruation, or seeing menstruation as gross), women do not simply internalize dominant norms from their interactions with larger social institutions (e.g., schools, health and medical services, prison), but instead they "respond creatively to these norms and generate their own views" (85). The cultural history of menstruation and the body may suggest ambivalent attitudes towards menstrual blood; however, menstruation is also a source of knowledge, resistance, and connection to oneself and others (Fingerson 94). The following section examines how the interaction between menstruation and *OITNB*'s comedic form positions menstruation and menstrual blood as metaphors for the intractable feminine, which, thereby, challenges imperatives for feminine comportment tied to women's regulation and management of their menstruating bodies.

Menses Madness: OITNB and the Unruly Feminine

OITNB's fictional account of prison and women prisoners' experiences examines menstruation within the necropolitical world of Litchfield penitentiary. As Zoey K. Jones suggests, prison is a place where inmates are marked as worthy of civil, social, political, and sometimes even biological death: "their bodies are and are not theirs; their exclusion from the social sphere defines the worlds both inside and outside of prison, and prisoners regularly suffer the violence of being made less-than-human" (142). As incarcerated women, the inmates are constructed as nonwomen—not real, not worthy, and not feminine. Although this status complicates the women's management of their menses by preventing them from being as "clean" as they would be outside prison, it also enables them to breech the menstrual mandate of shame, silence, and secrecy—something that *OITNB* highlights through comedy. As a comedy-drama, *OITNB* plays with the inherent polysemic nature of humour and irony (Palmer qtd. in Swink 16). According to Davis Murray, "comedic texts are particularly ambiguous and open to interpretation because humour is frequently predicated on disrupting expectations or playing with conceptual inconsistences, leading to *dramatically* different interpretations of the same content" (qtd. in Swink 16-17). In its engagement with menstruation, *OITNB* functions as a "double text" (Walker 31). The series addresses popular stereotypes about menstruation and menstruating bodies in order to humorously challenge and critique these very assumptions (Walker qtd. in Lauzen 109). A prime example is in the season-one episode "Tall Men With Feelings" when Piper Chapman (Taylor Schilling) confronts correctional officer Luschek for making an insensitive joke about suicide less than twenty-four hours after a deceased inmate (who had reportedly hanged herself) was found. Responding to Piper's retort, Luschek snaps, "Jesus Christ. You having your red dot special? Communists in your funhouse? Crimson tide?" Luschek's euphemisms are meant to silence and dismiss Piper, relegating her emotional needs to her being premenstrual. At the same time, however, Luschek's preference for euphemisms ironically calls attention to the very thing he is attempting to dismiss—that is, both Piper and, by extension, her menstruating body. Even though Luschek's euphemisms are intended to silence Piper, they also emphasize her position as an uncontrollable and unmanageable woman: she is unruly because she menstruates and because she challenges Luschek's authority.

As the scene continues, Piper (who is clearly annoyed by Luschek's dismissal of her needs) indignantly quips, "By all means, attribute my legitimate feelings of sadness to menses." Piper's use of the medically correct term "menses" is meant once again to challenge Luschek's authority, along with his preference for euphemisms in delegitimizing and dismissing her emotional needs. However, as a medically correct term, "menses" is seen as a snootier and a more pretentious word—snooty like Piper, who in her comment tacitly reveals the social and cultural expectations for feminine decorum. This difference is not lost on either Luschek or the other inmates who are also present for this exchange. In disbelief, Nicky Nichols (Natasha Lyonne) disapprovingly asks Piper "Did you really just say 'menses'?" before Luschek interjects with an emphatic "That's gross." Thus, in an ironic twist, Piper is subsequently made fun of along with Luschek's preference for euphemisms, as her character becomes a tacit critique of white, upper-middle class privilege through this scene's comedic engagement with menstruation.

A similar exchange occurs in the season-two episode "Take a Break from Your Values," in which Piper actively mobilizes premenstrual stereotypes to avoid punitive measures. In this scene, Piper receives some unfavourable news over the phone, and in her frustration, she slams the receiver down before banging her hands repeatedly against the wall. Correctional officer Charles Ford (Germar Terrell Gardner) witnesses Piper's outburst and sternly reminds Piper that the phone is federal property. Still fuming, Piper interrupts Ford with a lackluster comeback: "You're federal property!" Unimpressed by Piper's insubordination, Ford takes out his notepad and proceeds to write Piper a "shot"—a disciplinary slip given to inmates for behavioural infractions. Panicked, Piper apologizes profusely but to no avail, but then she exclaims, "Menses! It's menses madness!" Ford stops and responds with a resounding "Ew" before letting Piper go scot-free.

Although correctional officers are responsible for supervising and managing the inmates' behaviour, Piper's attribution of her outburst to feeling premenstrual enables her to circumvent disciplinary action. Piper's menstruating body exonerates her from responsibility for her inappropriate behaviour; it is not Piper that is acting out of turn but rather her leaky, open, and unruly body—a body that must be appropriately contained, regulated, and managed (Ussher 50). Ironically, Ford's intervention is to do just that: to discipline and control Piper's behaviour. However, because standards of feminine decorum are contingent upon women's self-policing of their menstruating bodies, only Piper can be made responsible for her outburst, not Ford. In other words, Piper's attribution of her outburst to menses ironically positions her as the only person who can appropriately negotiate and control her menstruating body, even though this attribution simultaneously absolves her from being entirely responsible for her disorderly behaviour. Thus, although Piper's comical deployment of premenstrual discourses reinforces common stereotypes that silence and dismiss women's emotional needs, it is a conscious tactic (unbeknownst to Ford) that enables her to avoid being reprimanded. Piper evokes normative understandings of femininity (specifically, the idea that good women ought to appropriately contain and control their bodies), but she ultimately challenges these assumptions by embracing her leaky and disruptive body in her evasion of disciplinary action.

In addition to *OITNB*'s engagement with the double text of humour and irony, menstrual blood and fluid are neither concealed nor shamefully denied; rather, they are humorously displayed and emphasized. An example is in the pilot episode "I Wasn't Ready" when Piper (who is at the time still new to prison life) receives a bloodied tampon in her food after unintentionally insulting Red's (Kate Mulgrew) cooking. (Red is a fellow inmate and also the prison's cook). In this scene, Piper joins the other inmates for breakfast in Litchfield's cafeteria. Seated at a table, she peels away the tinfoil covering her food to reveal an unmistakeable tampon string dangling out from inside her sandwich. Upon seeing this, Piper lifts the top slice of bread from her sandwich to reveal a medium close-up shot of a bloodied tampon. The shot immediately cuts to Piper's horrified reaction and then to the other inmates, who are more amused, if only mildly repulsed, than anything:

Morello: Oh. Oh? What did you do?

Nicky: She insulted the food in front of Red.

Morello: Oh jeez. I don't think you're gonna be eating for a while.

DeMarco: Put it away! I'm enjoying menopause very much, thank you.

Morello: You gotta figure out how to make things right with Red.

Piper's tampon sandwich is a classic cafeteria prank—though a particularly aggressive and shocking one—as menstrual blood is used to pit Red and Piper against each other. Although correctional officers can reprimand the women for such public acts of aggression (the bloodied tampon is served to Piper in broad daylight, and it becomes a central plot point in the following episode), the women choose to navigate this conflict without involving those who are in positions of authority. As Morello subtly implies to Piper, "snitching" to a correctional officer will likely make her current situation even more unbearable. (Piper does eventually make things right with Red, offering a makeshift lotion to help relieve Red's notable back pain—a concoction that requires Piper to comically suffer chewing through several spicy jalapeños for their anti-inflammatory properties.) Thus, although correctional officers may be responsible for the supervision, safety, and security of inmates, menstrual blood shows how the women can establish their own system for dealing with conflicts exceeding the limits of their incarceration. Ironically, however, the women are still incarcerated; they are ultimately subject to the authority of Litchfield's correctional officers, despite their ability to outsmart the guards in this instance.

Even in the absence of blood, references to menstruation and menstruating bodies are everywhere. Maxi pads and tampons—items meant to discretely absorb and dispose of blood—occupy a peripheral yet pervasive presence in the series. For instance, in the pilot episode bundles of maxi pads are depicted lying around the women's communal bunks. In addition to being used for their intended purpose, maxi pads (since they are available for free and in large quantities)[1] are also repurposed by the women into items Litchfield fails to provide. For example, Piper uses maxi pads as a pair of shower shoes after she cannot purchase them from the prison's commissary due to a processing delay upon her arrival at Litchfield. Additionally, many inmates use maxi pads to clean their bunks to meet the prison's high inspection standards, or they use them in combination with either a hair tie or an elastic band to make makeshift eye- and facemasks. (The harsh lighting in the prison, as well as the smell of the inmates' flatulence from eating poor quality food, limits the women's available sleeping hours.) Cardboard tampon applicators are also repurposed to conceal contraband, such as cigarettes.

The women's repurposing of menstrual products comes to a head when Litchfield experiences a menstrual product shortage in season four. In this episode "We'll Always Have Baltimore," the women's struggle to access menstrual supplies forces some of the inmates to barter for items in the black market economy or to create makeshift menstrual products out of everyday objects. For example, one inmate humorously creates a tampon out of an empty toilet paper roll and a toothbrush; another comically contemplates using a plastic medicine cup in place of a proper menstrual cup, and another dismantles her maxi pad sleep mask for its original intended use: to absorb and dispose of menstrual blood. By emphasizing the unavoidable and unavoidably intimate needs of the menstruating body, the episode highlights the complex nature of institutionalized violence—punishment for which the inmates are seen as deserving, given their status as incarcerated nonwomen. This violence is exemplified through concerns of the body that have historically been coded as feminine, such as the deeming of menstrual products as inessential. Thus, by narrativizing the private details of menstruation through comedy, *OITNB* emphasizes the connection between seemingly small-scale women's concerns and larger patterns of institutionalized gender oppression as well as the women's possibilities for agency under such conditions.

The ubiquity of maxi pads and tampons, as well as the women's repurposing and incorporation of them into many other aspects of their lives in prison, serve as referents for women's disruptive bodies within the prison that contains them. Not only do these items signify the very thing they are supposed to discretely contain (i.e., menstrual blood), even in their unbloodied state, they also disclose how the women inmates can exceed the disciplinary and regulatory limits of incarceration. The women's humorous repurposing of products in place of other items Litchfield fails to supply as well as their frank and unfiltered discussions about their periods construct them as defiant figures. In other words, these referents for menstruation perform a kind of metaphoric volatility. Their presence challenges normative understandings of femininity that are contingent upon women's concealment and the regulation of their menstruating bodies, which makes visible how the women of Litchfield cannot be contained.

Difference and the Unruly Feminine

Negotiating menstruation through comedy, humour, and irony, *OITNB* posits alternative accounts of femininity through unruly feminine figures. Litchfield physically confines and controls women's bodies through disciplinary measures and forms of surveillance. Yet the prison functions as an equalizer of sorts, as many of the women inmates share the fate of not only their bodies (i.e., they bleed) but also their physical containment within communal prison space. Despite this shared fate, *OITNB* avoids flattening difference and idealizing sameness among women (which are exclusionary practices) by portraying multifaced experiences of menstruation. The series' menstruation narratives prominently feature working-class and women of colour, and, in doing so, they challenge essentialism by demonstrating how identity is located in the intimate, embodied aspects of daily life. An example is how Litchfield's menstrual product shortage affects some women more deeply than others. In the episode "We'll Always Have Baltimore," Litchfield must operate on the same budget for inessentials, such as maxi pads, despite a recent influx of over one hundred new inmates.[2] In one scene, the women are depicted in an exceptionally long line to receive maxi pads from the prison's medical depot. Upon hearing that the depot has run out of pads, the remaining women become frustrated. One woman of colour, Alison Abdullah (Amanda Stephen), scoffs at the fact that her "baby box" has been deemed inessential, while another, Reema Pell (Mugga), laments the unaffordable cost of tampons at $10 per box, given the inmates' hourly wage of $0.10. The depot manager shrugs indifferently before Gina sarcastically quips, "What are we supposed to do? Use toilet paper?" Witnessing the commotion, another woman of colour, Michelle Carreras (Arianda Fernandez), boasts about having enough tampons for her upcoming cycle if she only uses one per day, despite (perhaps unknowingly) placing herself at risk of toxic shock syndrome. The shot then pans to recovering meth addict Angie Rice (Julie Lake), who in overhearing the preceding conversation, comically shares with her friend Leanne Taylor (Emma Myles) that she used to substitute dinosaur just-add-water sponges for kids for tampons outside prison. Leanne laughs, as Angie continues, "It was really fun! 'Cause it was like, 'Oh, I wonder what this will be? Oh! Brontosaurus Rex! Covered in baby blood!'"

The above scene underscores the connection between lived experience and identity through menstrual blood; the women's management of their menstruating bodies is not just tied to imperatives for feminine comportment; it is also contingent upon their status as nonwomen both in- and outside of prison. Angie's humorous anecdote in particular highlights how the various methods used by the women to attend to their periods are incongruous with the social and cultural expectations for how women ought to manage their cycles. Although her remark about using "Brontosaurs Rex" just-add-water sponges suggests a resourcefulness that will help her negotiate the supply deficit, it also calls attention to her socioeconomic status outside of prison, given her inability to afford or access tampons. At the same time, Angie's status as an incarcerated nonwoman enables her to transgress the menstrual mandate of shame, silence, and secrecy. Her working-class status may contribute to her marginalization outside prison (her use of tampon substitutes reflects a failure to adequately manage her menstruating body); however, within the context of Litchfield, this resourcefulness becomes a highly valued mode of knowledge, resistance, and connection to oneself and others (Fingerson 93-94). Thus, the irony in Angie's statement emphasizes the extent to which she, as a working-class woman, is already positioned outside of normative femininity. Angie's anecdote is comical precisely because her methods for previously managing her cycle are anything but discrete or ladylike.

The menstrual supply scarcity, in combination with the high price of tampons sold at the prison's commissary, also forces predominately working-class women of colour to resort to outlandish methods to manage their cycles. In the episode "We'll Always Have Baltimore," Alison, Michelle, and Reema are depicted commiserating in the bathroom as they MacGyver makeshift menstrual products out of everyday items. Reema pushes a wad of towel through an empty paper toilet roll with the back of her toothbrush, while Alison sighs, "Bye-bye, sleep mask. Time to meet my snizz" and removes the elastic band from her maxi pad. Beside her, Michelle closely examines a plastic medicine cup and asks: "Think it'll stay in?" Alison looks over before cautioning, "Just don't lose it up there; that could get serious." Shortly after, Cindy Hayes (Adrienne C. Moore), one of the few women able to afford tampons from the prison's commissary, walks in to use the toilet, tampon in hand. Reema jeers "Well, la-di-da. Little Miss One Percent herself" before Michelle asks, "What are you charging for one of those?" Cindy pauses, smirks, and then says: "Five dollars." The women immediately protest, and even though Michelle attempts to negotiate with Cindy, it does not take long for her and the other women to realize that Cindy's priority is making a profit in the prison's black market economy rather than helping her fellow inmates.[3]

As this scene illustrates, Litchfield's inadequate supply of menstrual products implicates many, if not all, menstruating women; however, humour and irony reveal the specificities of how the inmates can manage their bodies—a process that is contingent upon each woman's proximity in relation to the norm. The working-class women of colour mobilize their menstruating bodies in different ways than Cindy, who is instead focused on profiting from the economic misfortune of others. Rather than conceal their bodies, Aliso, Michelle, and Reema draw on the specificities of their experiences to respond to the supply deficit as a source of pride and resourcefulness; they use menstruation as a tool for making valuable connections and sharing improvisational skills in commiserating about their shared circumstance (Fingerson 93-94).

OITNB's menstruation narratives not only represent women who belong to "demographics classically marked for death" but also demonstrate the consequences of marginalization (Jones 142-143). Through the inmates' comical and unconventional methods for negotiating Litchfield's menstrual supply shortage, menstruation shows how women's abilities to appropriately regulate and manage their menstruating bodies are necessarily classed and raced; the women may share the fate to bleed in prison, but class and race continue to constitute the regimes of intelligibility through which menstruating bodies are materially mediated.

Conclusion

OITNB exemplifies the complex ways in which menstruation is made discursive through comedy, humour, and irony. From its depiction of menstrual products to its engagement with the inherent polysemic nature of comedy, *OITNB* creates referents for menstruation that posit alternative modes of femininity. Menstruation makes visible women's leaky, open, and excessive bodies, and, by extension, it constructs the inmates as unruly feminine figures. In other words, it is through their permeable and menstruating bodies that the women can exceed the limits of their incarceration—whether that is through the repurposing of menstrual products into items Litchfield fails to supply or through evading disciplinary action from correctional officers who are in positions of power and authority. Thus, in *OITNB*'s engagement with menstruation, comedic conventions are integral to highlighting not only how women's incongruous behaviours and actions challenge normative femininity but also how identity is located within the intimate, embodied aspects of daily life.

Endnote

1. Although earlier seasons of *OITNB* depict an abundance of menstrual products, with the women inmates repurposing sanitary napkins and tampons for a number of miscellaneous goods, press accounts detail the struggles of actual incarcerated women to acquire menstrual product, which serves as a counterpoint to the series' fictionalization of prison life. These accounts emphasize how women's access to menstrual supplies in prison continues to be limited, even after the emergence of new legislation supporting menstrual product access (as for example the Canadian government's elimination of its national goods and service tax on menstrual products in 2015, and the passing of a set of bills in New York City guaranteeing free menstrual supplies to women in public schools, homeless shelters, and prisons in 2016) (see Greenberg 2017). Responding to this shifting sociocultural context, *OITNB* later offered a narrativized account of these struggles in the season-four episode "We'll Always Have Baltimore."

2. Litchfield is acquired by the Management & Correction Corporation and becomes a privatized institution.

3. This scene escalates the conflict between Alison and Cindy, who are both depicted earlier in the episode arguing over Cindy's unwillingness to lend Alison a tampon, despite having the economic

means to do so. Although Cindy is also a woman of colour, her financial stability is conflated with her recent conversion to Judaism: she refers to her ability to afford tampons as simply being "chosen." This intersection between class and religion is further explored during the women's exchange in the bathroom scene when Reema refers to Cindy's charging of interest for tampons as something "her people do." Although Cindy accuses Reema for propagating hate speech, she in the same breath rejects Alison's request to barter and states: "The only language this Jew here speak [sic] is cold hard cash. You see, it's okay when I say it."

Works Cited

Chrisler, Joan C. "Leaks, Lumps, and Lines: Stigma and Women's Bodies." *Psychology of Women Quarterly*, vol. 35, no. 2, 2011, pp. 202-214.

Davis, Murray. *What's So Funny?: The Comic Conception of Culture and Society*. Chicago University Press, 1993.

Erchull, Mindy J. "Distancing Through Objectification? Depictions of Women's Bodies in Menstrual Product Advertisements." *Sex Roles*, vol. 68, no. 32, 2013, pp. 32-40.

Fahs, Breanne. "Sex During Menstruation: Race, Sexual Identity, and Women's Accounts of Pleasure and Disgust." *Feminism & Psychology*, vol. 21, no. 2, 2011, pp. 155-178.

Fingerson, Laura. *Girls in Power: Gender, Body, and Menstruation in Adolescence*. State University of New York Press, 2006.

Greenberg, Zoe. "In Jail, Pads and Tampons as Bargaining Chips." *The New York Times*, April 20, 2017.

www.nytimes.com/2017/04/20/nyregion/pads-tampons-new-york-womens-prisons.html. Accessed 1 Mar. 2019.

"I Wasn't Ready." *Orange Is the New Black*, created by Jenji Kohan, performance by Taylor Schilling, season 1, episode 1, Netflix, 11 July 2013.

Jackson, Theresa E., and Rachel J. Falmagne. "Women Wearing White: Discourses of Menstruation and the Experience of Menarche." *Feminism & Psychology*, vol. 23, no. 3, 2013, pp. 379-398.

Johnston-Robledo, Ingrid, and Margaret L. Stubbs. "Positioning Periods: Menstruation in Social Context: An Introduction to a Special Issue." *Sex Roles,* vol. 68, 2013, pp. 1-8.

Johnston-Robledo, Ingrid, and Joan C. Chrisler. "The Menstrual Mark: Menstruation as Social Stigma." *Sex Roles,* vol. 68, 2013, pp. 9-18.

Jones, Zoey K. "Pleasure and Power Behind Bars: Resisting Necropower with Sexuality." *Feminist Perspectives on Orange Is the New Black: Thirteen Critical Essays,* edited by April Kalogeropoulos Householder and Adrienne Trier-Bieniek, McFarland, 2016.

Kerman, Piper. *Orange Is the New Black: My Year in a Women's Prison.* Spiegel & Grau, 2010.

Kissling, Elizabeth A. "Bleeding Out Loud: Communication about Menstruation." *Feminism & Psychology,* vol. 6, no. 4, 1996, pp. 481-504.

Kotthoff, Helga. "Gender and Humor: The State of the Art." *Journal of Pragmatics,* vol. 38, no. 1, 2006, pp. 4-25.

Lauzen, Martha. "The Funny Business of Being Tina Fey: Constructing a (Feminist) Comedy Icon." *Feminist Media Studies,* vol. 14, no. 1, 2014, pp. 106-117.

Merrill, Lisa. "Feminist Humor: Rebellious and Self-Affirming." *Women's Studies,* vol. 15, 1988, pp. 271-280.

Mizejewski, Linda. *Pretty/Funny.* University of Texas Press, 2014.

"Riot FOMO." *Orange Is the New Black,* created by Jenji Kohan, performances by Abigail Savage, Matt Peters, and Laura Gómez, season 5, episode 1, Netflix, 9 June 2017.

Rowe, Kathleen. "Rosanne: Unruly Woman as Domestic Goddess." *Screen,* vol. 31, no. 4, 1990, pp. 408-419.

Rowe, Kathleen. *The Unruly Woman: Gender and Genres of Laughter.* University of Texas Press, 1995.

Russo, Mary. "Female Grotesques: Carnival and Theory." *Feminist Studies / Critical Studies,* edited by Teresa de Lauretis, Indiana University Press, 1986, pp. 213-229.

Swink, Robyn Stacia. "Lemony Liz and Likeable Leslie: Audience Understandings of Feminism, Comedy, and Gender in Women-Led Television Comedies." *Feminist Media Studies*, vol. 17, no. 1, 2017, pp. 14-28.

"Take a Break from Your Values." *Orange Is the New Black,* created by Jenji Kohan, performances by Taylor Schilling and Germar Terrell Gardner, season 2, episode 11, Netflix, 6 June 2014

"Tall Men With Feelings." *Orange Is the New Black,* created by Jenji Kohan, performances by Taylor Schilling and Matt Peters, season 1, episode 11, Netflix, 11 July 2013.

Ussher, Jane M. *Managing the Monstrous Feminine: Regulating the Reproductive Body.* Routledge, 2006.

Wagner, Kristen Anderson. "'Have Women a Sense of Humour?' Comedy and Femininity in Early Twentieth-Century Film." *The Velvet Light Trap*, vol. 68, 2011, pp. 35-46.

Walker, Nancy. *A Very Serious Thing: Women's Humor and American Culture.* University of Minnesota Press, 1988.

"We'll Always Have Baltimore." *Orange Is the New Black,* created by Jenji Kohan, performances by Amanda Stephen, Abigail Savage, and Julie Lake, season 4, episode 5, Netflix, 17 June 2016.

Notes on the Contributors

Cayo Gamber is an associate professor of writing and women's, gender, and sexuality studies at the George Washington University. She publishes research on the ways the Holocaust is represented through museums, memorials, archival images, and artifacts. She also interrogates the role of popular culture in creating Western notions of girlhood and womanhood.

Claire Horn is a PhD candidate in law at Birkbeck University, where she is researching the legal and ethical implications of artificial womb technology. She is a graduate teaching assistant in criminology, and holds an MA from New York University and BA from McGill.

Berkeley Kaite has published on pornographic magazines (*Pornography and Difference,* Indiana University Press, 1995), the photography of Sally Mann (in *Mothering and Psychoanalysis,* Demeter, 2014), and the iconicity of Jacqueline Kennedy (*Celebrity Studies, Teorija in Praksa*), among others. She is an associate professor in the Department of English at McGill University.

Barbara Kutis is assistant professor of art history at Indiana University Southeast. Her research focuses on women, gender, domesticity, and parenting. Her current book project, forthcoming with Routledge, is titled *Artist-Parents in Contemporary Art: Gender, Identity, and Domesticity.* The book addresses artists' engagement with parenting, gender, and identity in their art.

Laura Helen Marks is a professor of practice in English at Tulane University. Her work on pornographic genre, adaptation, and neo-Victorian studies has appeared in *Sexualities, Phoebe, Salon, Porn Studies, Feminist Media Histories,* and *Porno Chic and the Sex Wars* (University of Massachusetts Press, 2016), and is forthcoming in *Cinema Journal.* Marks also contributes to the adult film oral history podcast *The Rialto*

Report. Her book, *Alice in Pornoland: Hardcore Encounters with the Victorian Gothic*, is forthcoming in 2018 with Illinois University Press.

Peter Ohlin has written extensively on the films of Ingmar Bergman as great modernist masterpieces, discussing, for example, the ways in which they treat the fact of the Holocaust and whether allegations about Bergman's youthful Nazi past can be seen in his films. His latest book is *Wordless Secrets. Ingmar Bergman's* Persona*: Modernist Crisis and Canonical Status* (Wales: Welsh Academic Press, 2011).

Katerina Symes is a PhD candidate in the Department of Communication Studies at Concordia University, Montreal, Canada. Her research is supported by the Social Sciences and Humanities Research Council of Canada (SSHRC) and has been published in the *Oxford Handbook of Feminist Theory* and *Feminist Media Studies*.

Kasia Van Schaik is a doctoral student at McGill University and the fiction editor of the Quebec Writers' Federation Journal, *Carte Blanche*. Kasia's writing has appeared in *Electric Literature, The Los Angeles Review of Books, The Best Canadian Poetry Anthology* (2015), *CBC Books, Prism International* and elsewhere. Her first collection of poetry, *Sea Burial Laws According to Country*, was published in 2018. Kasia lives in Montreal.

Deepest appreciation to
Demeter's monthly Donors

DEMETER

Daughters
Muna Saleh
Summer Cunningham
Rebecca Bromwich
Tatjana Takseva
Kerri Kearney
Debbie Byrd
Laurie Kruk
Fionna Green
Tanya Cassidy
Vicki Noble
Bridget Boland

Sisters
Kirsten Goa
Amber Kinser
Nicole Willey
Regina Edwards